Heroines & Heroes

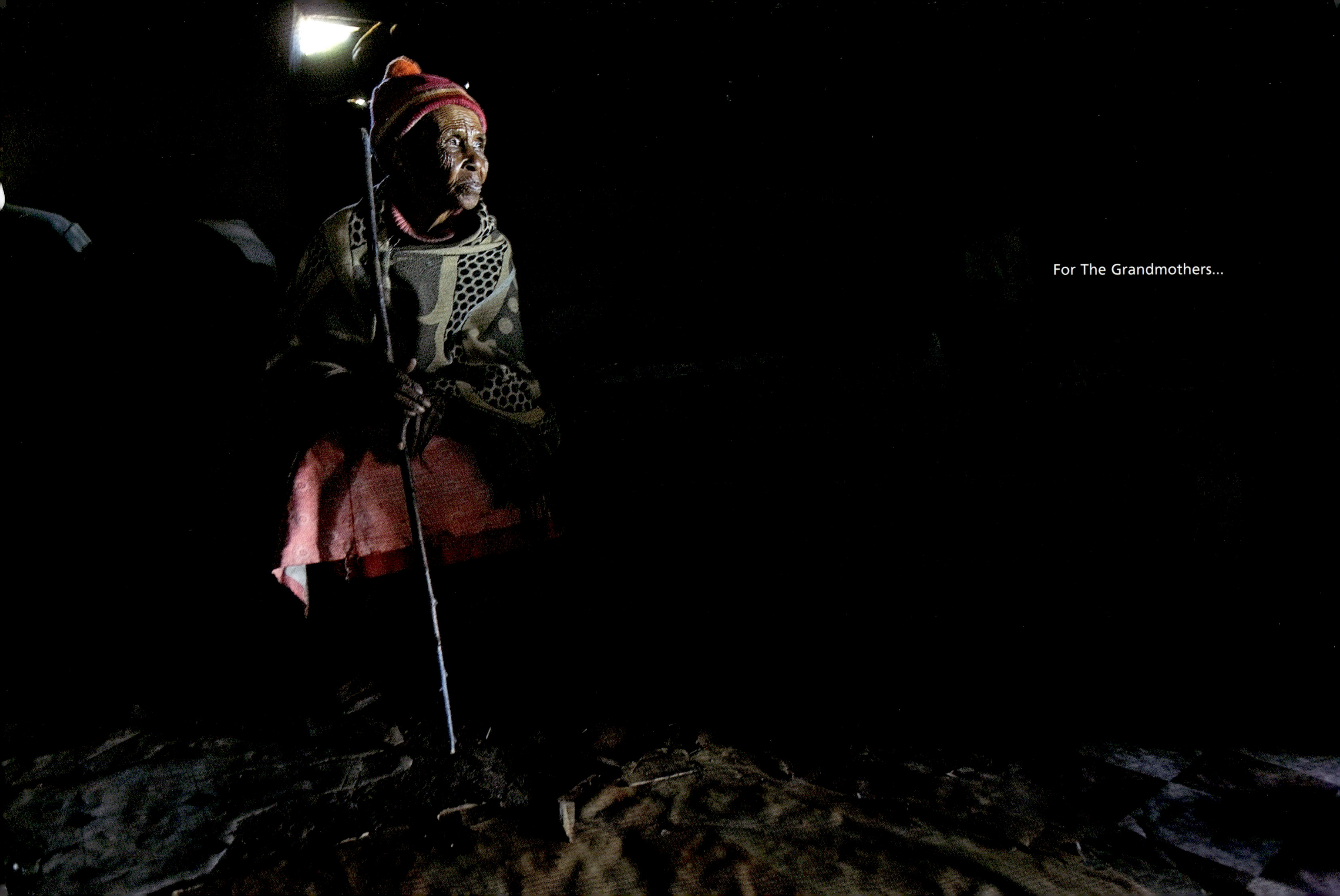
For The Grandmothers...

Heroines & Heroes
Hope, HIV and Africa

by Steve Simon

CHARTA

Concept
Steve Simon

Design
Daniela Meda

Editorial Coordination
Filomena Moscatelli

Copyediting
Charles Gute

Copywriting and Press Office
Silvia Palombi Arte&Mostre, Milano

Web Design and Online Promotion
Barbara Bonacina

Cover
A group of children pose for a photograph
in Leribe, Lesotho. An estimated 12 million
children under the age of 17 (just under
10% of all children) living in sub-Saharan
Africa have lost one or both parents to AIDS.

Back Cover
Children near Maseru, Lesoth, persevere
against the wind and rain after school

© 2006
Edizioni Charta, Milano

© Steve Simon for his photographs

© The authors for their texts

All rights reserved
ISBN 88-8158-610-X

Edizioni Charta
via della Moscova, 27
20121 Milano
Tel. +39-026598098/026598200
Fax +39-026598577
e-mail: edcharta@tin.it
www.chartaartbooks.it

Printed in Italy

To see more work by Steve Simon, go to
www.stevesimonphoto.com

Contents

It must be understood, without any hint of heady romanticism, that Africa in the 1950s and 1960s, when I was most impressionable, was a continent of vitality, growth and boundless expectation. It got into your blood, your viscera, your heart.

The bonds were not just durable, they were unbreakable. There was something intoxicating about an environment of such hope, anticipation, affection, energy, indomitability.

The Africa I knew was poor, but it wasn't staggering under the weight of oppression, disease and despair; it was absolutely certain that it could triumph over every exigency. There were countless health emergencies—polio, measles, malaria, malnutrition—but it never felt like Armageddon. In fact, life expectancy began to rise in the late 1960s, until the reversal induced by Structural Adjustment Programs on the one hand, and AIDS on the other.

And the people, the people everywhere, were so unbelievably kind; I had never encountered cultures so uniformly inclusive, gentle, decent, welcoming.

I was smitten for life.

You can understand, therefore, how painful it is to visit my beloved Africa under present-day circumstances. It's not just the ruinous economic and social decline, it's the ravaging of the pandemic; it's the way in which a communicable disease called AIDS has taken countries by the throat and reduced them to spectral caricatures of their former selves.

I have to say that the ongoing plight of Africa forces me to perpetual rage. It's all so unnecessary, so crazy that hundreds of millions of people should be thus abandoned.

From *Race Against Time*, Stephen Lewis
United Nations Special Envoy for HIV/AIDS in Africa

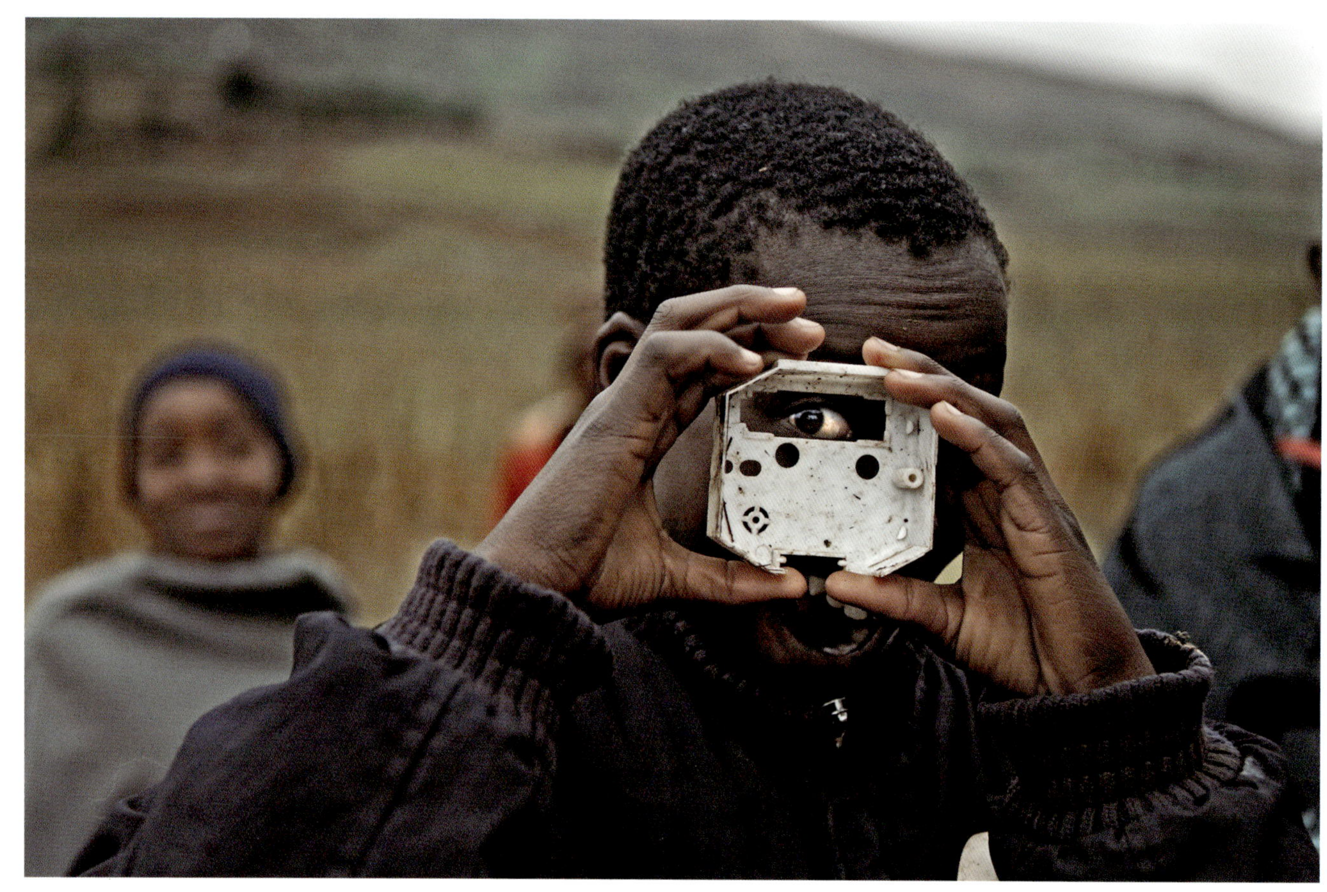

The more I travel and meet the people in Africa, the more questions I ask myself. What would my life be like if I had been born in Africa? How strong would I be? Would I have my sense of humor? Would I be optimistic? Could I care about others when my own life is such a struggle? Would I have my passion for photography?

In the Mountain Kingdom of Lesotho, a beautiful country of rolling hills and cold winters where 36% of the nearly two million people earn an average of less than $1 per day, survival is the mantra for most. There are few choices.

I ask myself these questions because the people I meet are just like me, or my family and friends. Alex is my age and he struck me as a wise man who would be a professor or businessman if life had worked out differently.

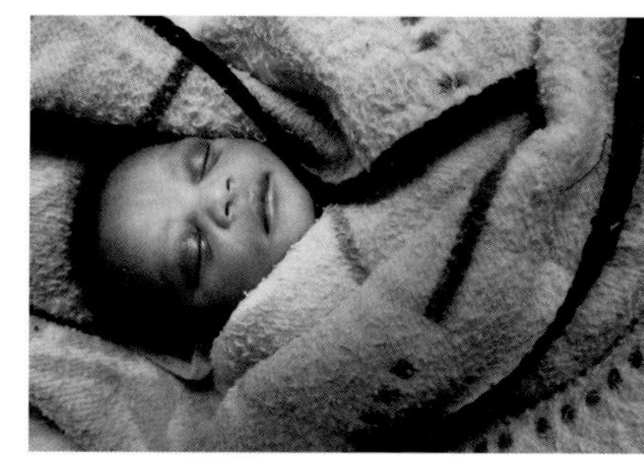

Instead, he worked in the mines for years and is now in the hospital with tuberculosis. He told me about his crystal-clear memory of the moment when all his dreams evaporated as a young boy, when his parents told him they could no longer afford his school fees. I felt again how fate works its way into all our lives.

This book is not about statistics; it is about people in the places I have traveled in Lesotho, Ethiopia, Zambia and Mozambique. Know that HIV prevalence rates and the massive numbers of people dying from AIDS are devastating. The word *pheello* is a Sesotho word meaning "perseverance." Persevere is what the heroines and heroes in the fight against AIDS do. The grandmothers, who have buried their own children and are now raising the grandchildren, even great-grandchildren, persevere. The orphans, having experienced a lifetime's worth of trauma in their brief time on earth, persevere. Caregivers, the medical teams and AIDS counselors, the volunteers and the patients themselves—many who have to endure unthinkable pain and neglect, as the brutal AIDS-related illnesses slowly take the life from their bodies—all continue the fight.

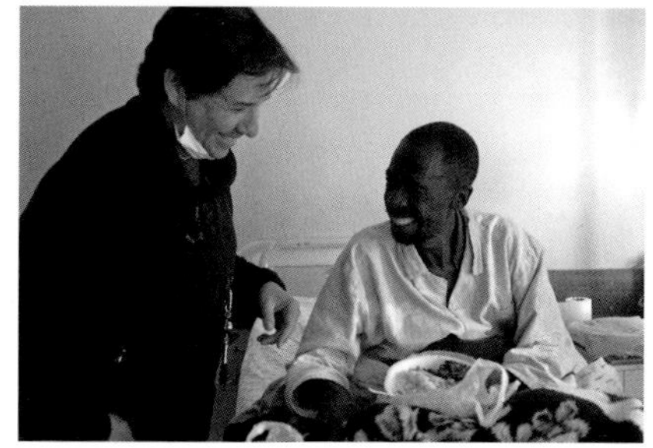

Fighting the pandemic of AIDS is a complex and layered problem, without easy or quick solutions. Millions of lives are at stake, and the fine people I have met while working on this book, many of whom are suffering a life of extreme poverty, are some of the brightest, wisest, funniest and most inspiring people I have ever known. They are the people you love in your own lives. They should not be ignored.

At the end of this book is a "Call To Action" section, with information on what you can do to help. In many places progress is being made, so let's keep our governments accountable and make sure we are giving what we should and doing what we can. We can make a difference.

Steve Simon

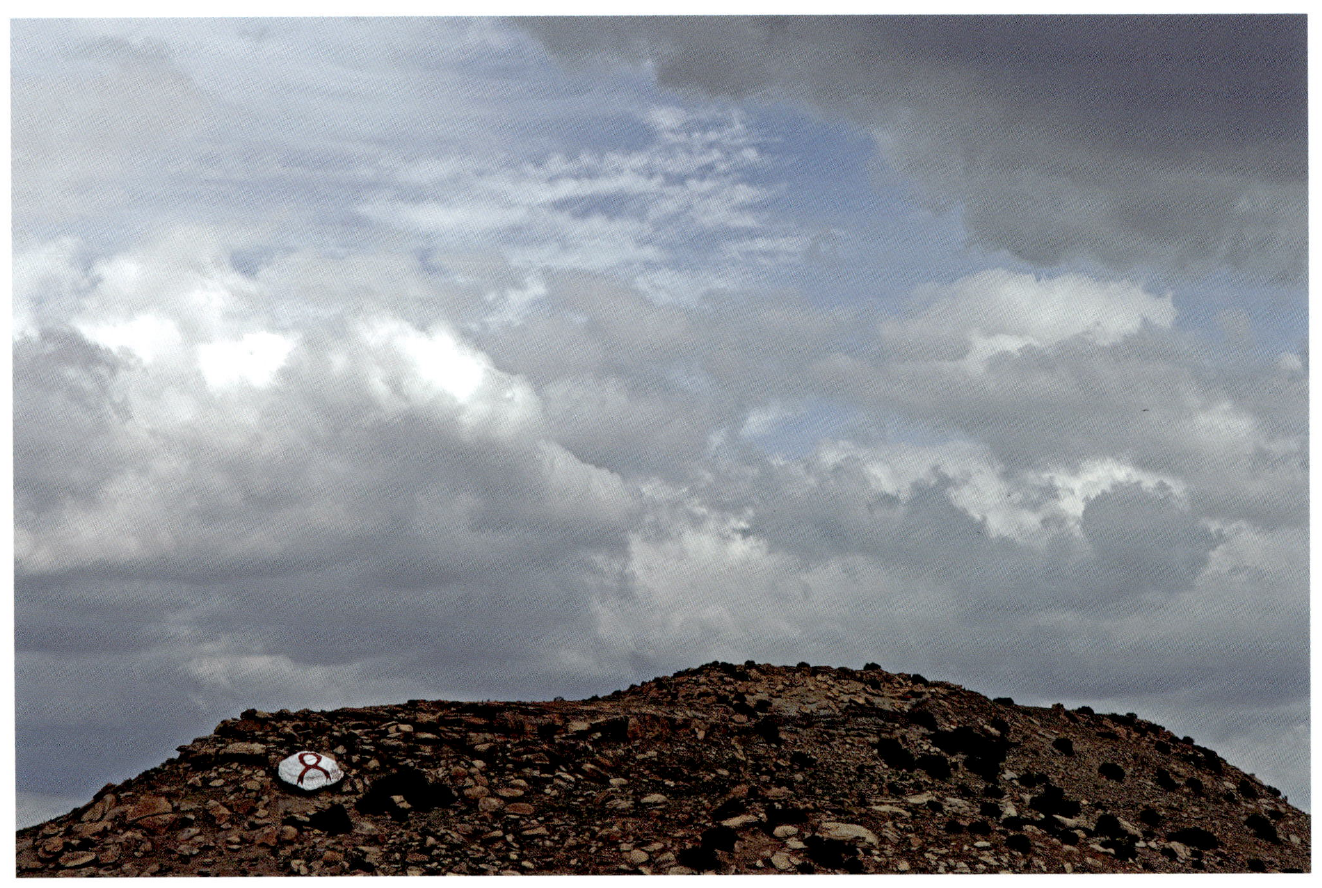

We need to educate the people about HIV and AIDS and how they should take care of themselves. Community education is moving very, very slowly, even though there has been much information on the radio and in the papers. Many people do not listen to the radio or read the papers. We need to educate students while they are still young, but not leave the parents behind, because they also need to be educated to keep their health and fight the stigma.

Stigma comes with tradition, and when it is emphasized that HIV is transmitted through sex, such talk of sex is a taboo in this country. One big problem is people who are afraid to get tested to see if they are HIV-positive or not, especially when they are very healthy. They are afraid because when people find out you are positive, you are an outcast. There are other misguided beliefs. Some people think the testing will make you positive. The testing itself!

Personally, I have lost many friends, and the disease has created many orphans with no one to take care of them. We have extended families but AIDS has separated us. Families can no longer or will no longer take care of their own.

We also lack facilities, and even though we now have the use of ARV drugs to extend life, we need to make them more available so people do not need to travel long distances to get them. Some people take the ARVs for the first six months and then stop. They say, "I'm better now," so there's no use in making the long journey to keep getting them.

We need to find a remedy for HIV and AIDS. We should be able to prevent it and treat it, but also be able to have our babies. Of course condoms are important to prevent HIV and AIDS, but are we going to be able to produce and have our own babies like our fathers did?

If we are not able to have children it means we are going nowhere. The nation to come won't have another generation. The people will be gone. All the beautiful houses will be empty because we will be dead, no one will be there. The parents will die and even the children will go; they will just vanish into thin air because of a lack of knowledge.

I have knowledge so I must pass it on to others and help. I believe in working together, moving forward together. At the end of the day, we can win.

Chief Joseph Tseea

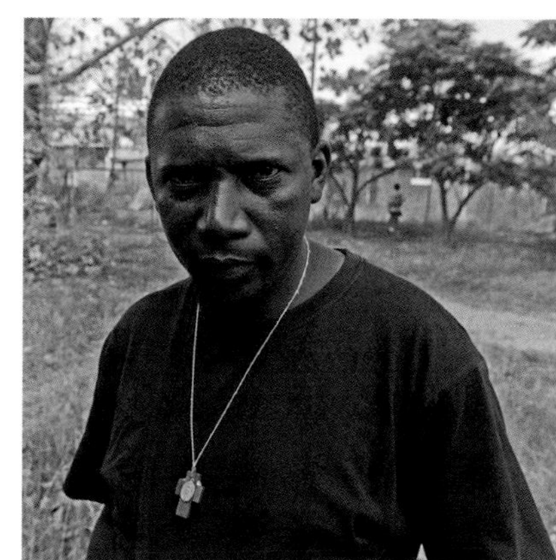

Chief Joseph Tseea from the village of Haramoabi, Lesotho. Teacher and Red Cross volunteer

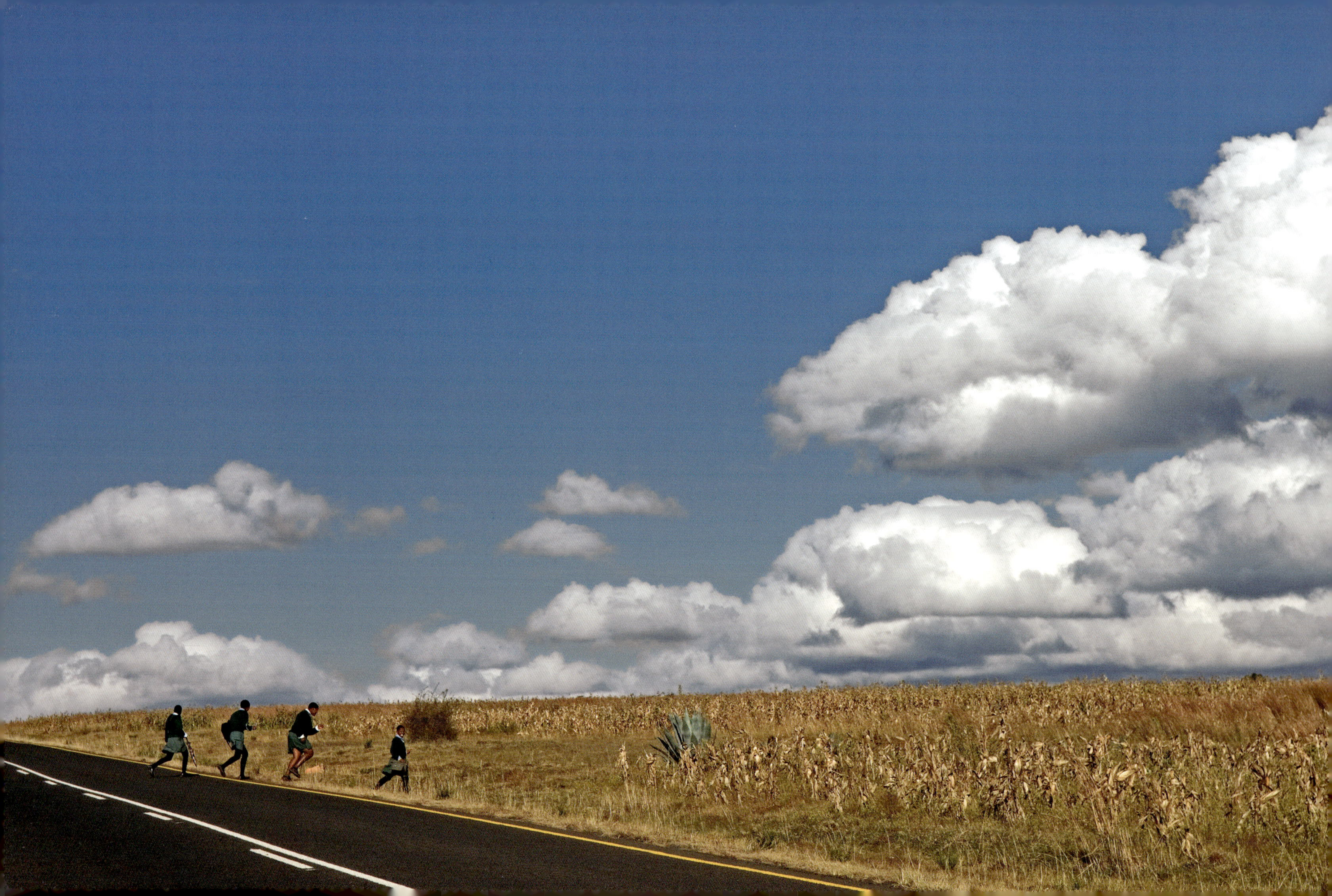

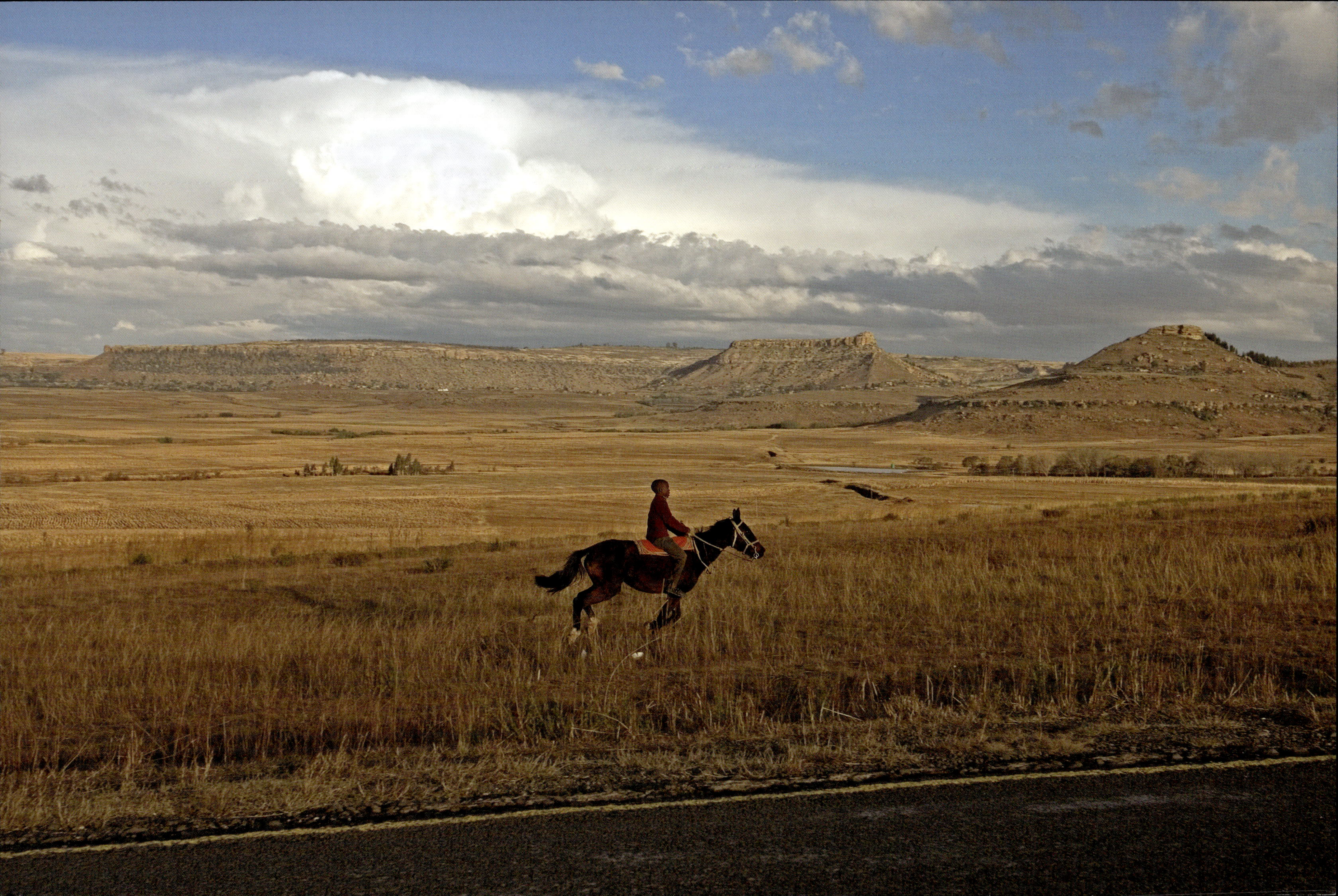

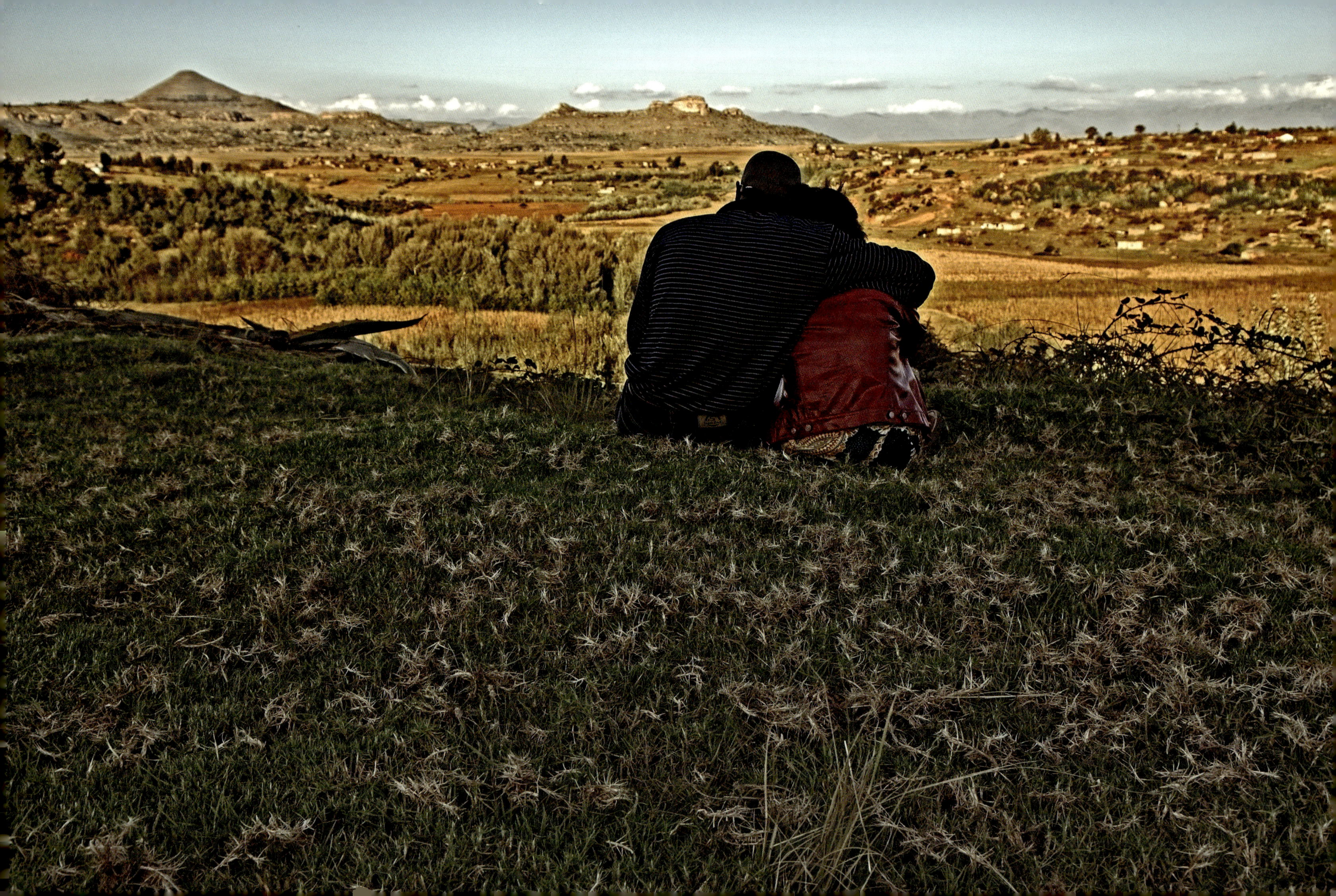

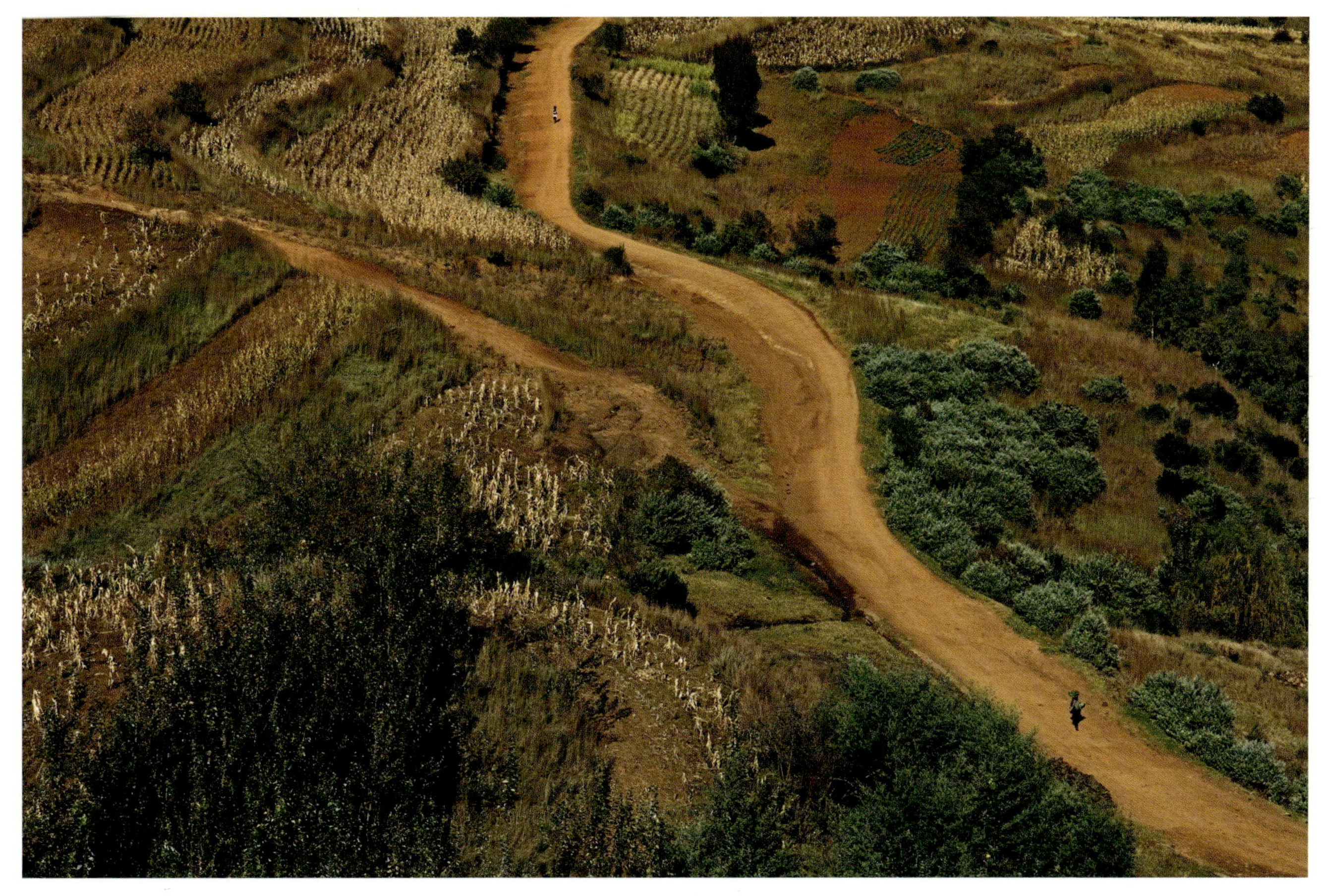

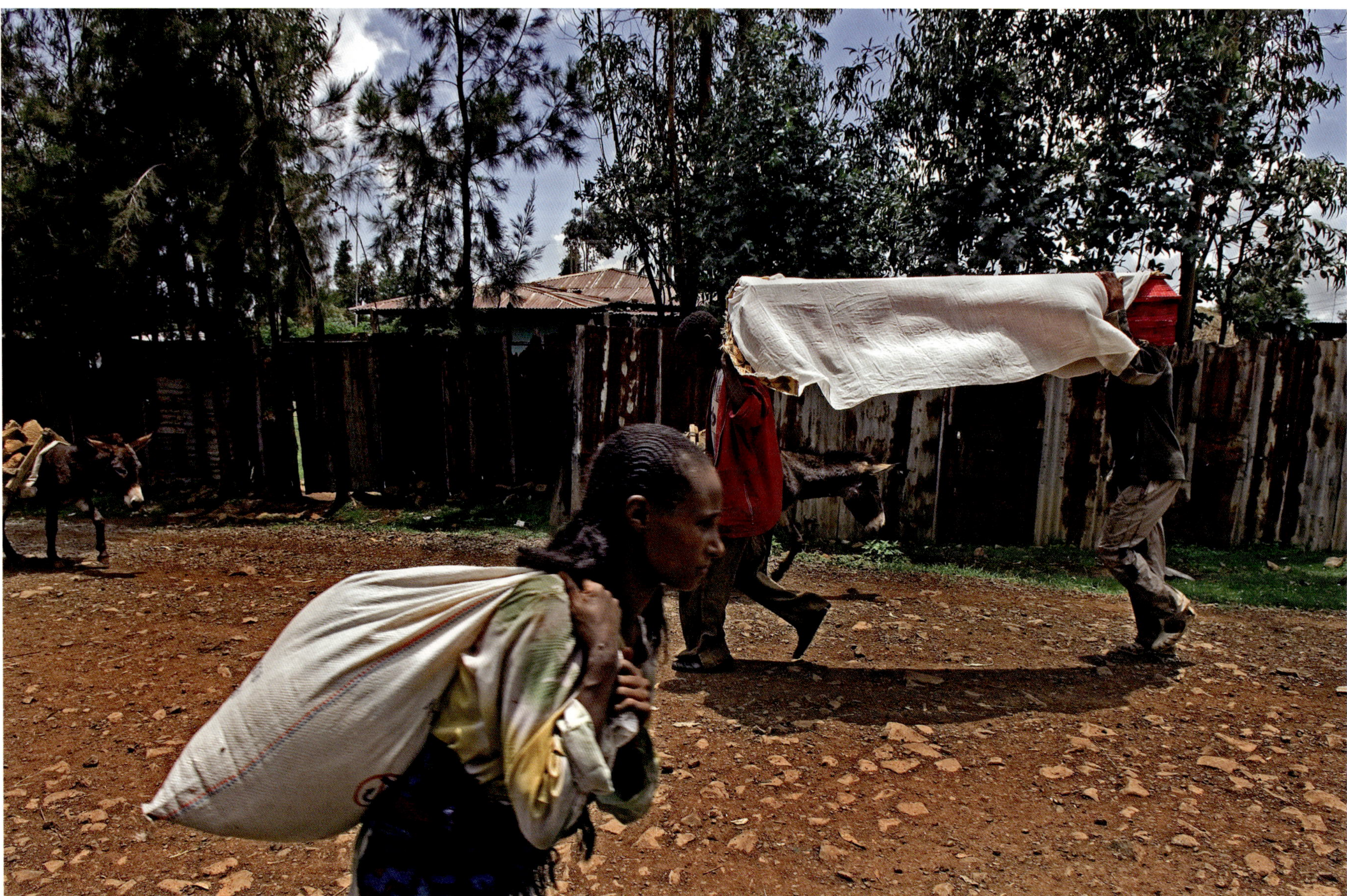

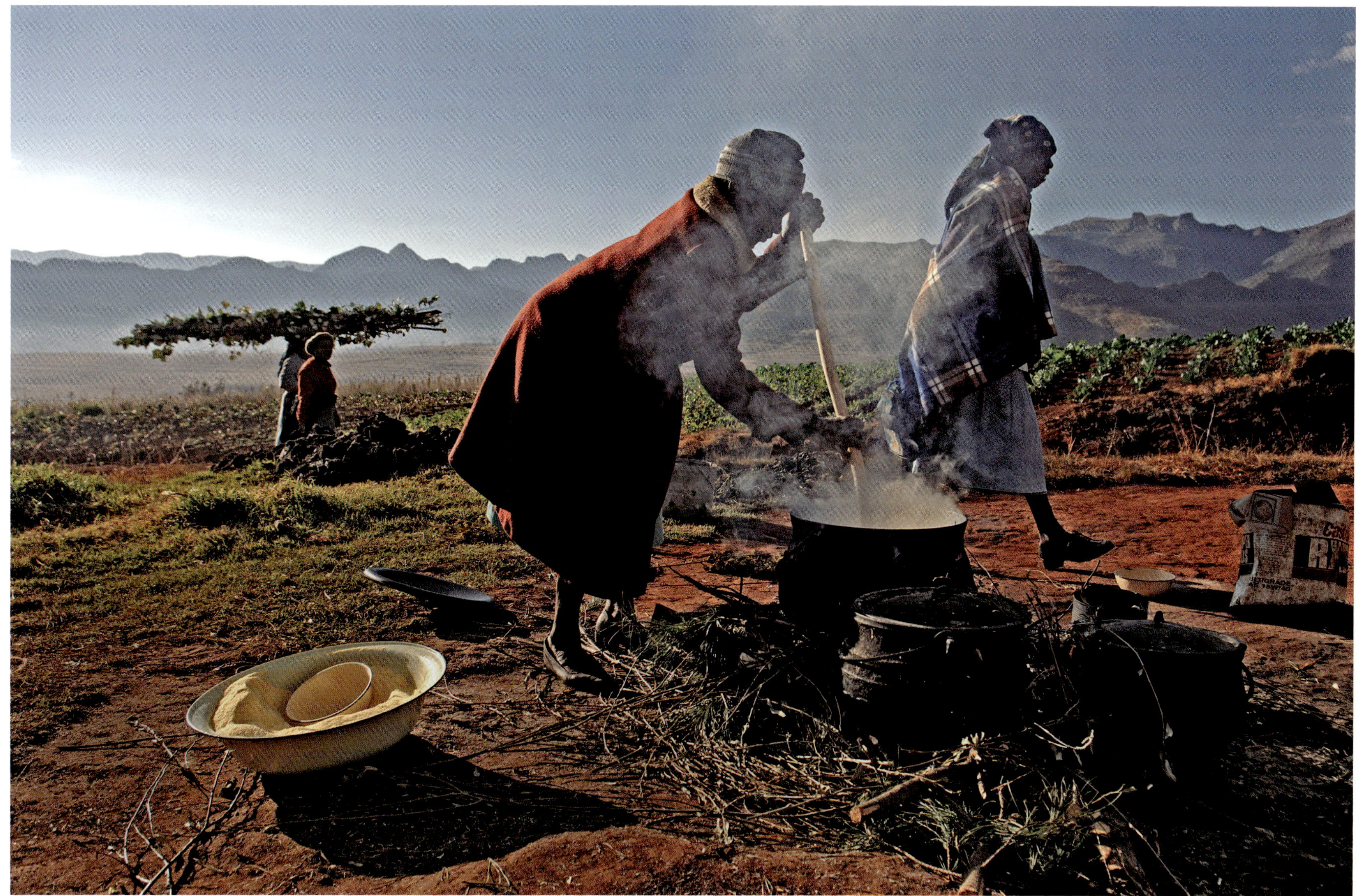

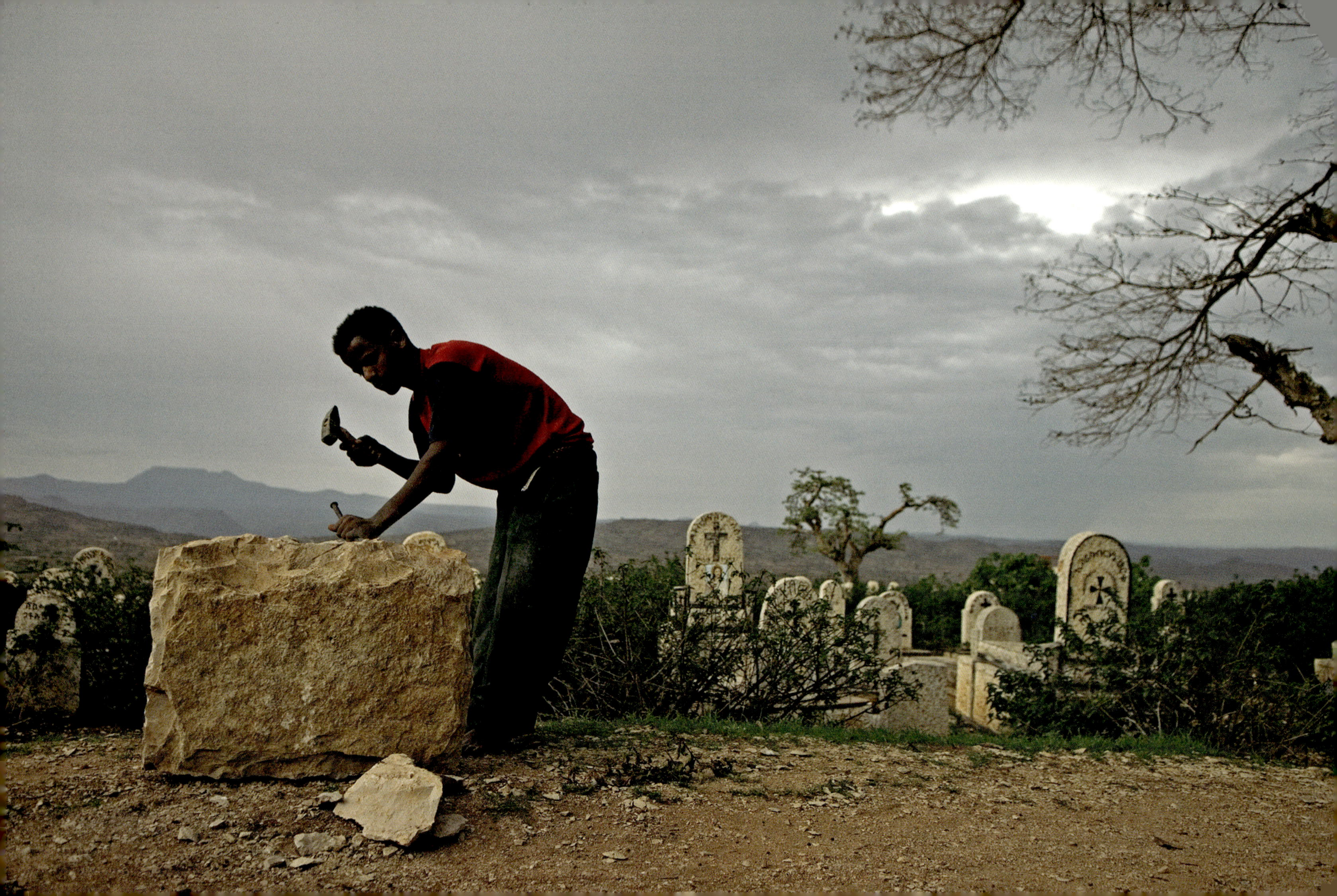

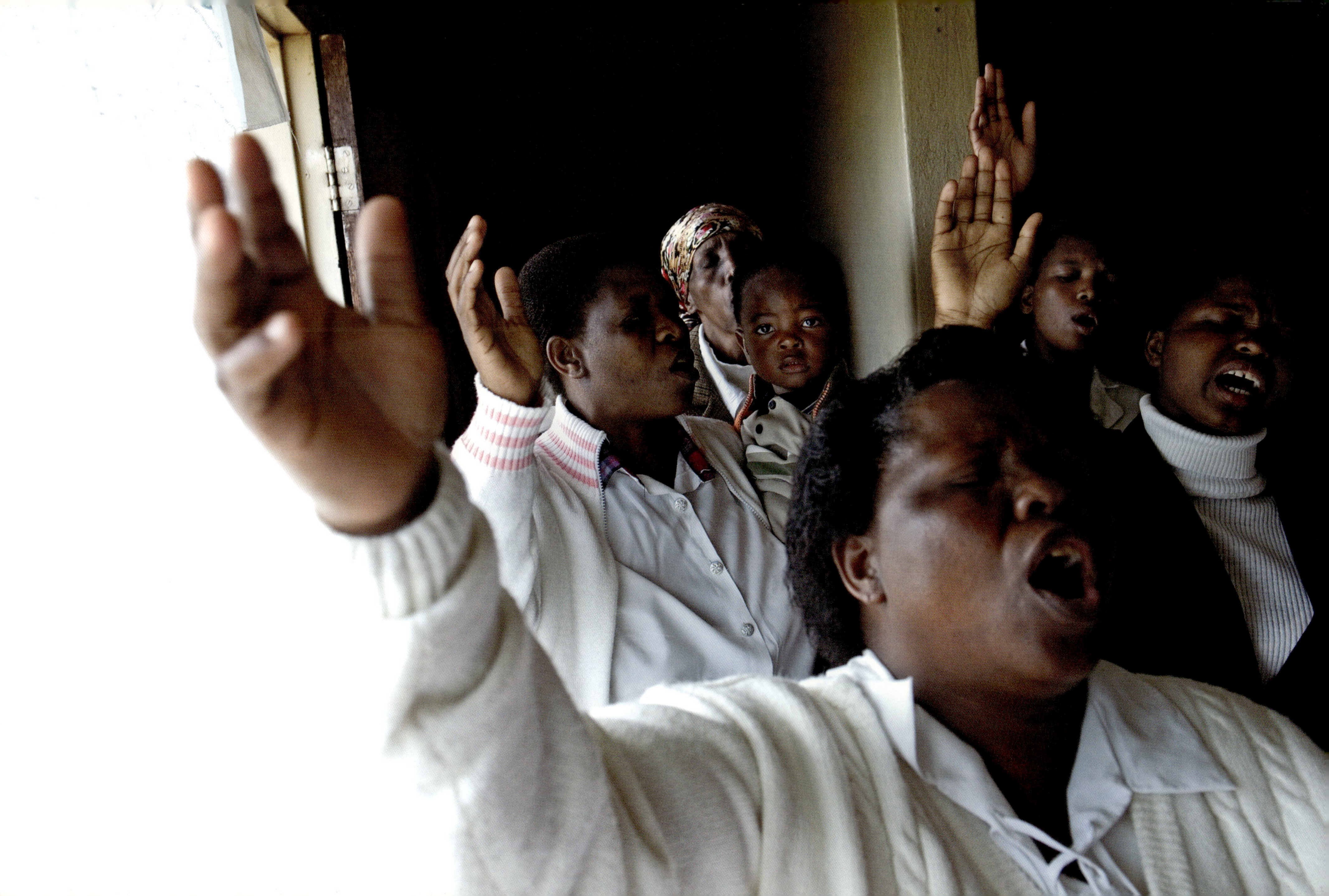

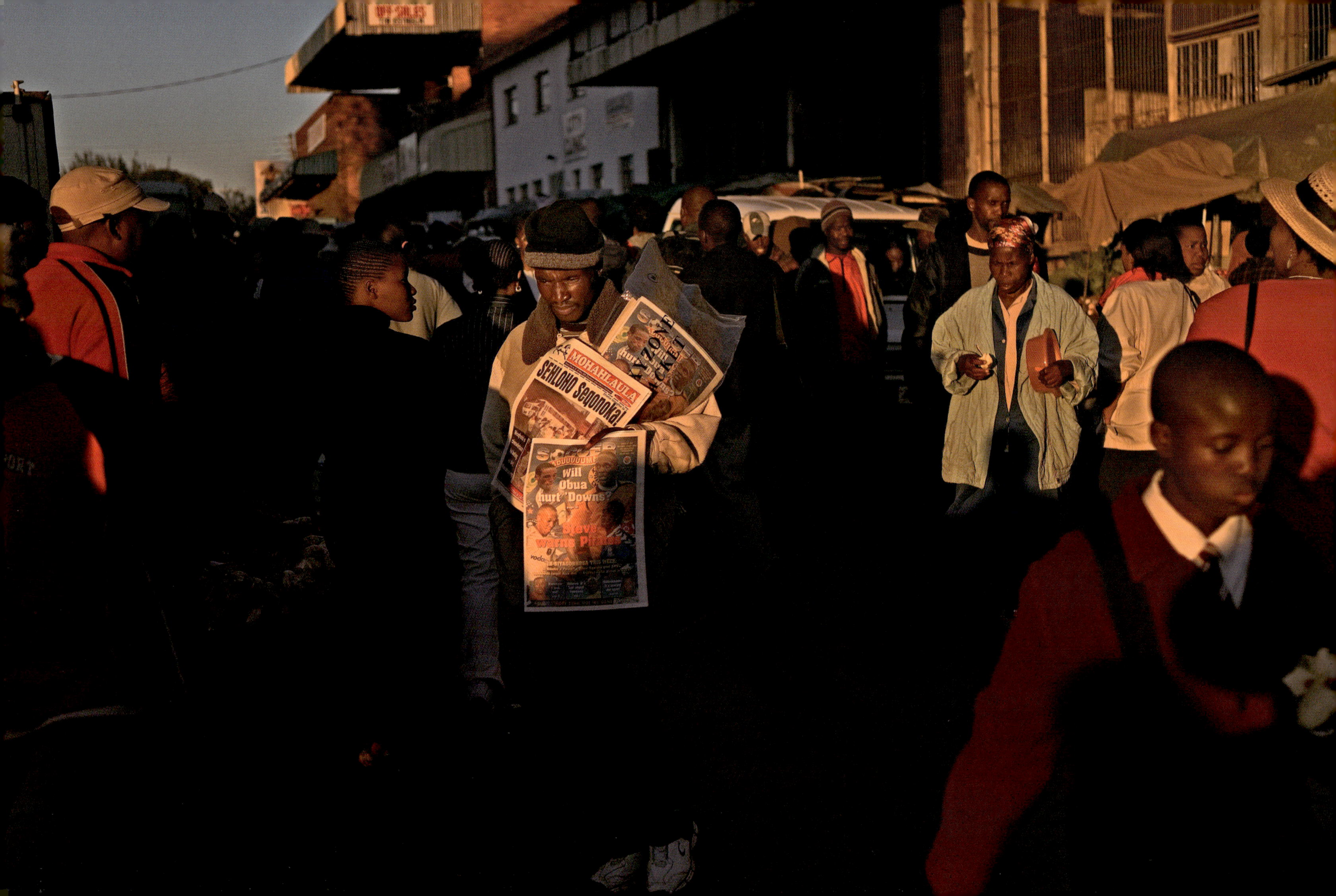
MOHAHLAULA
SEHLOHO Seqonoka!
SOCCER ZONE
Will Obua hurt 'Downs?
SOCCER
Will Obua hurt 'Downs?
Steve warns Pirates
voda

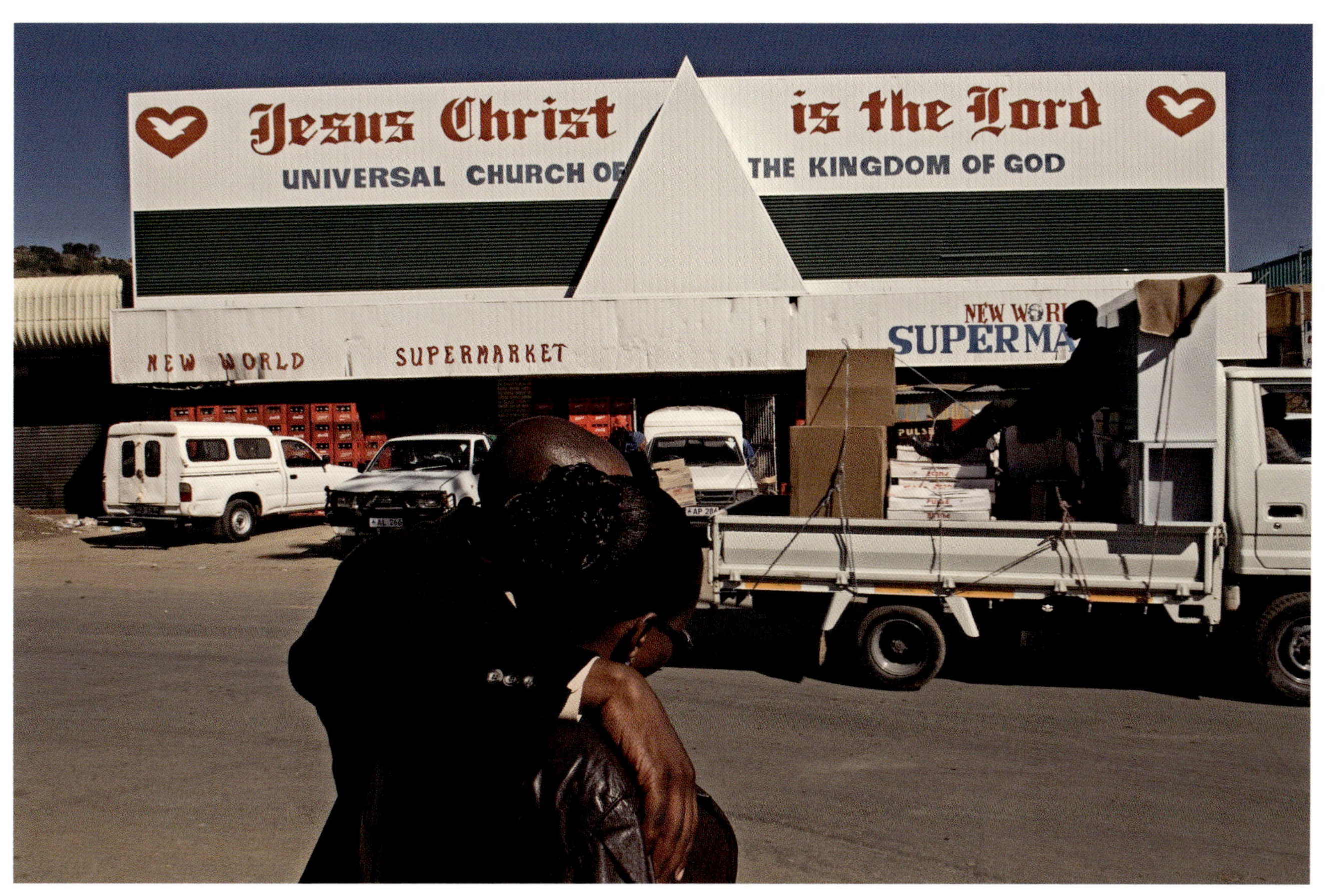

Jesus Christ   is the Lord
UNIVERSAL CHURCH OF THE KINGDOM OF GOD
NEW WORLD SUPERMARKET
NEW WORLD
SUPERMA

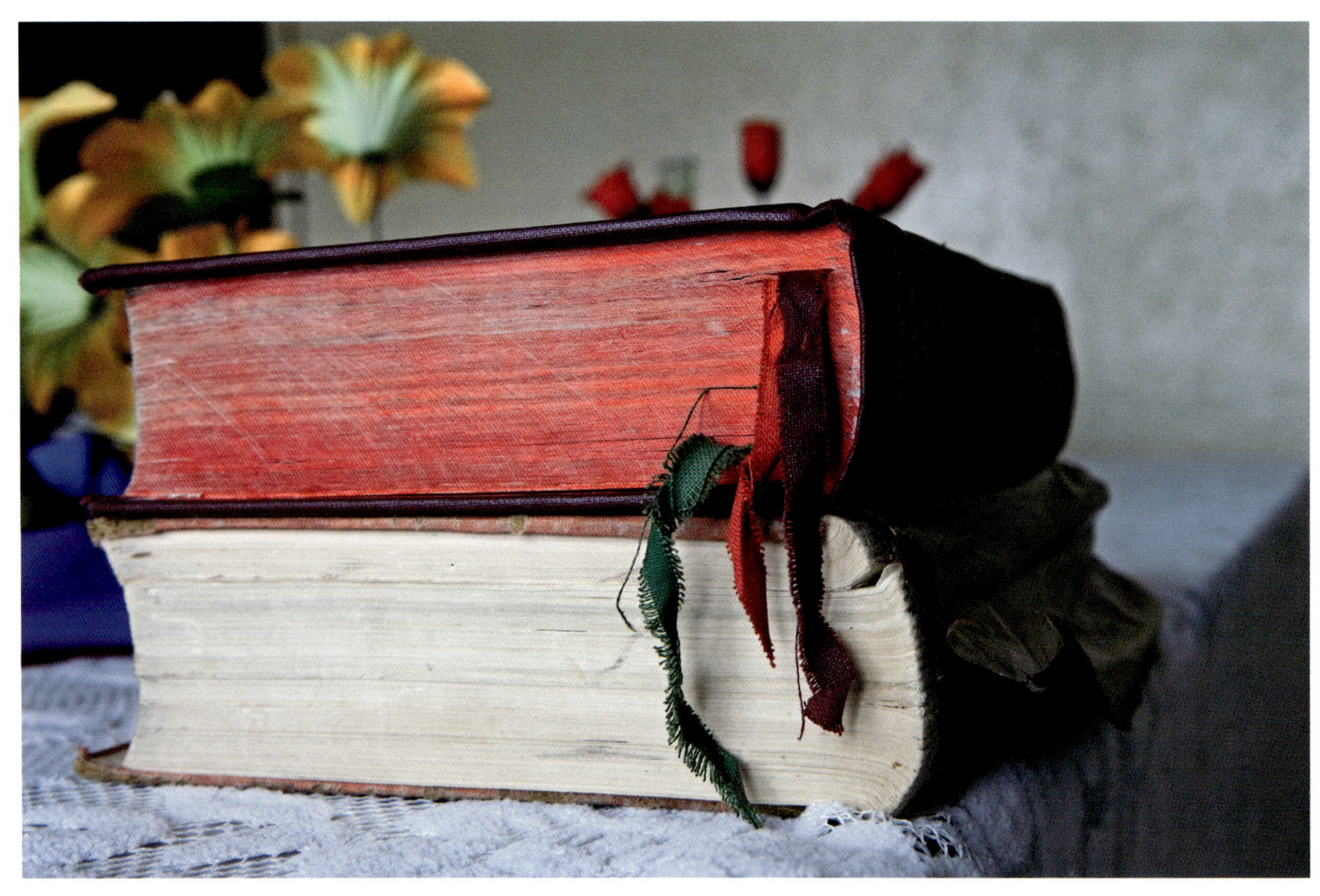

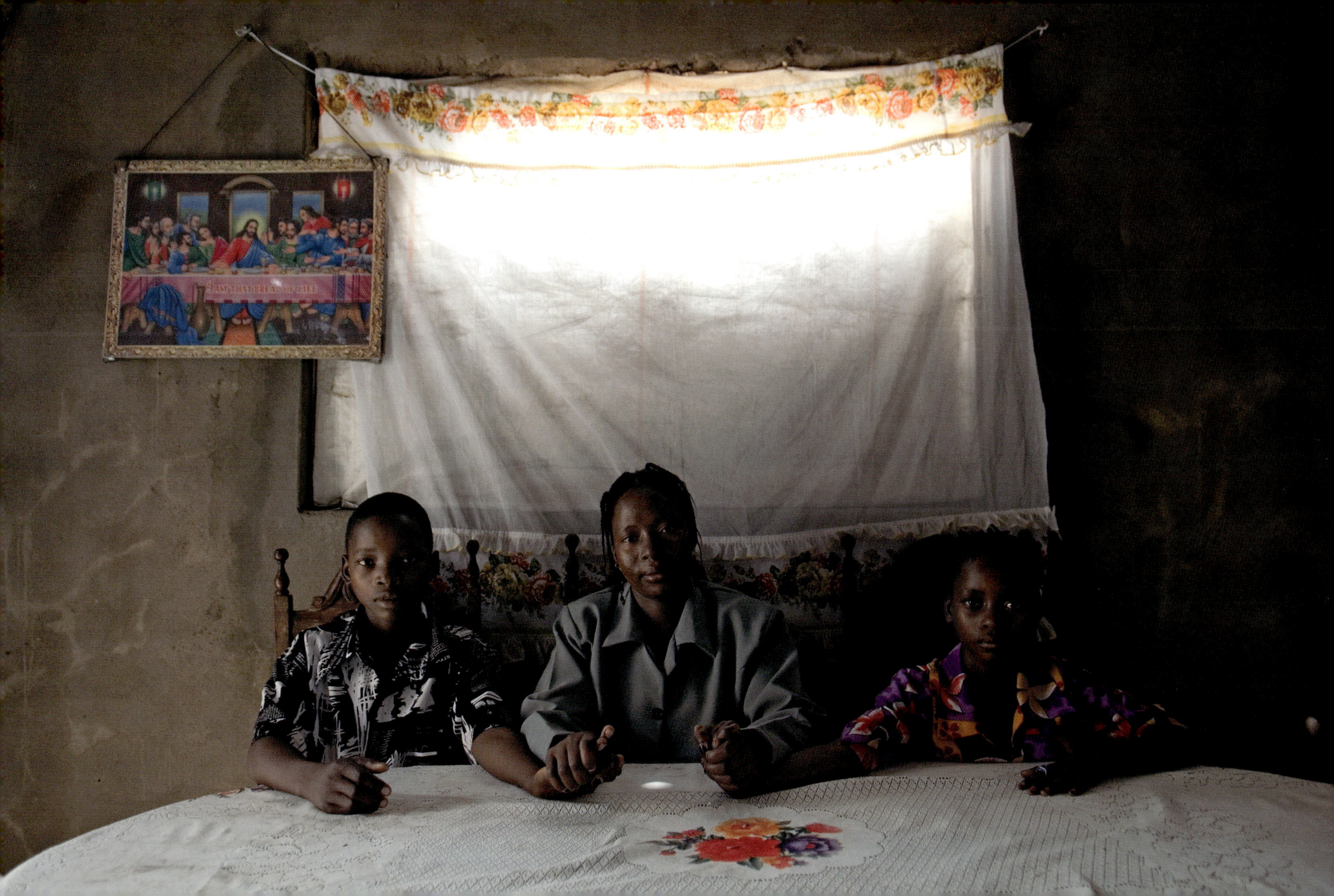

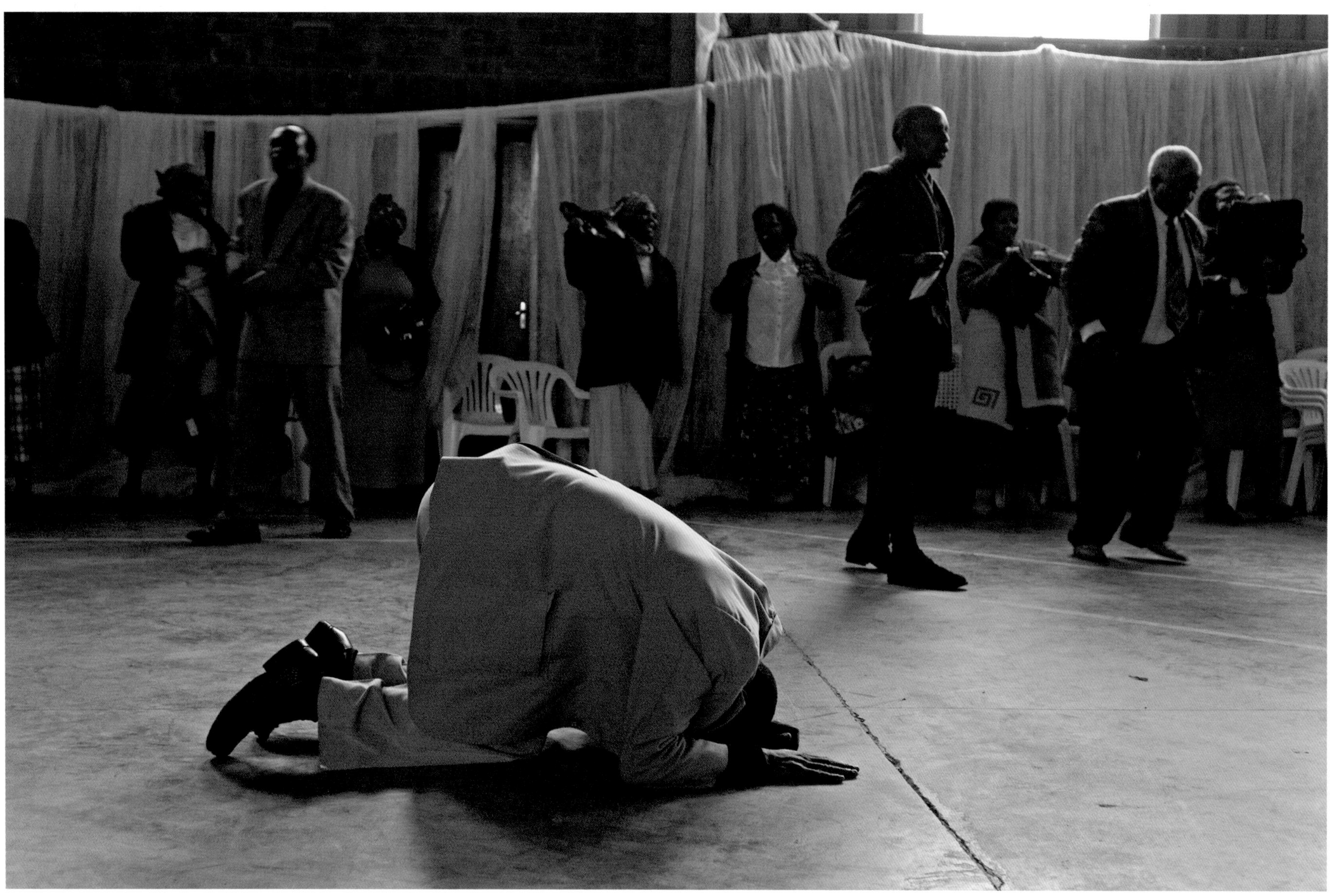

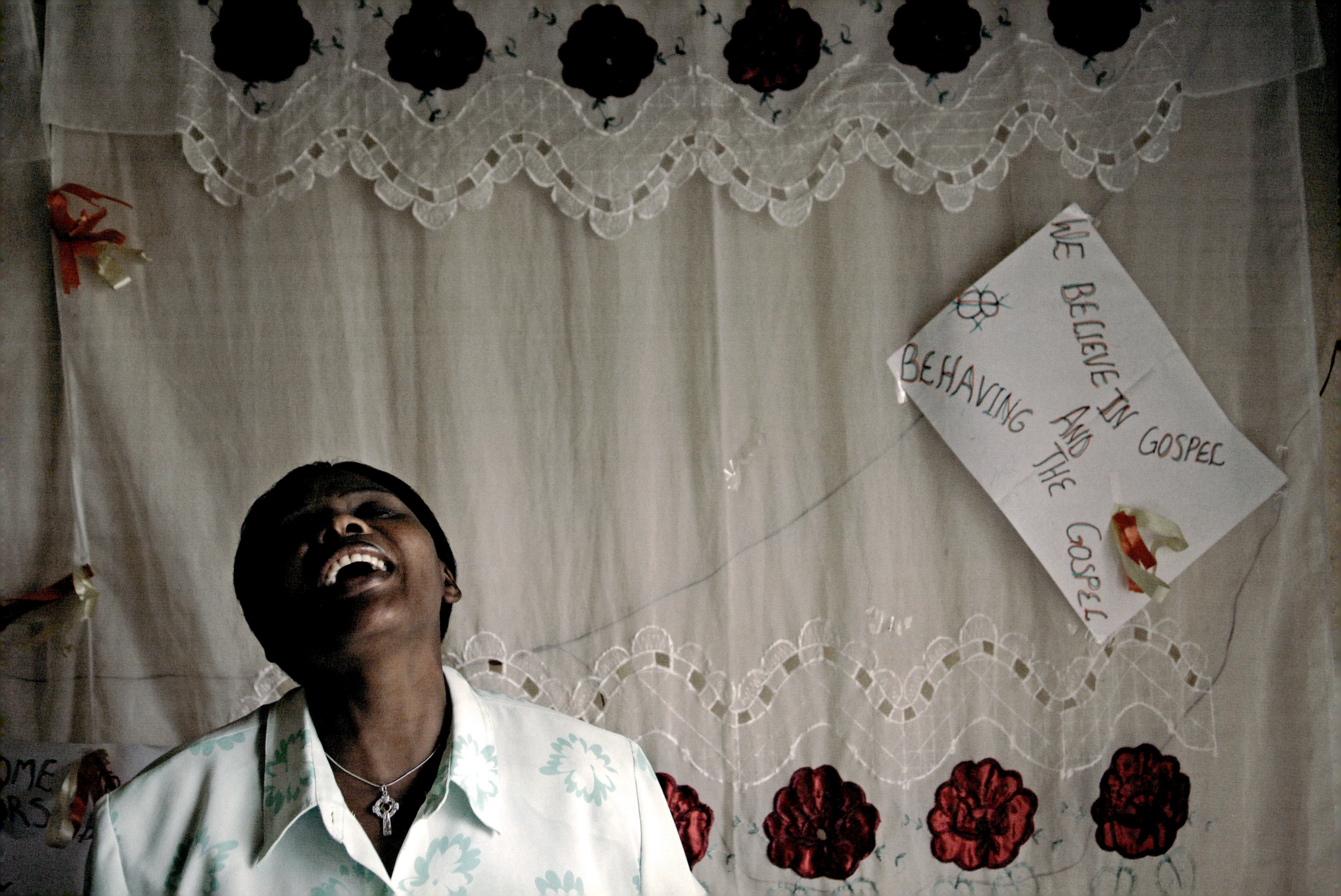
WE BELIEVE IN GOSPEL
BEHAVING AND THE GOSPEL

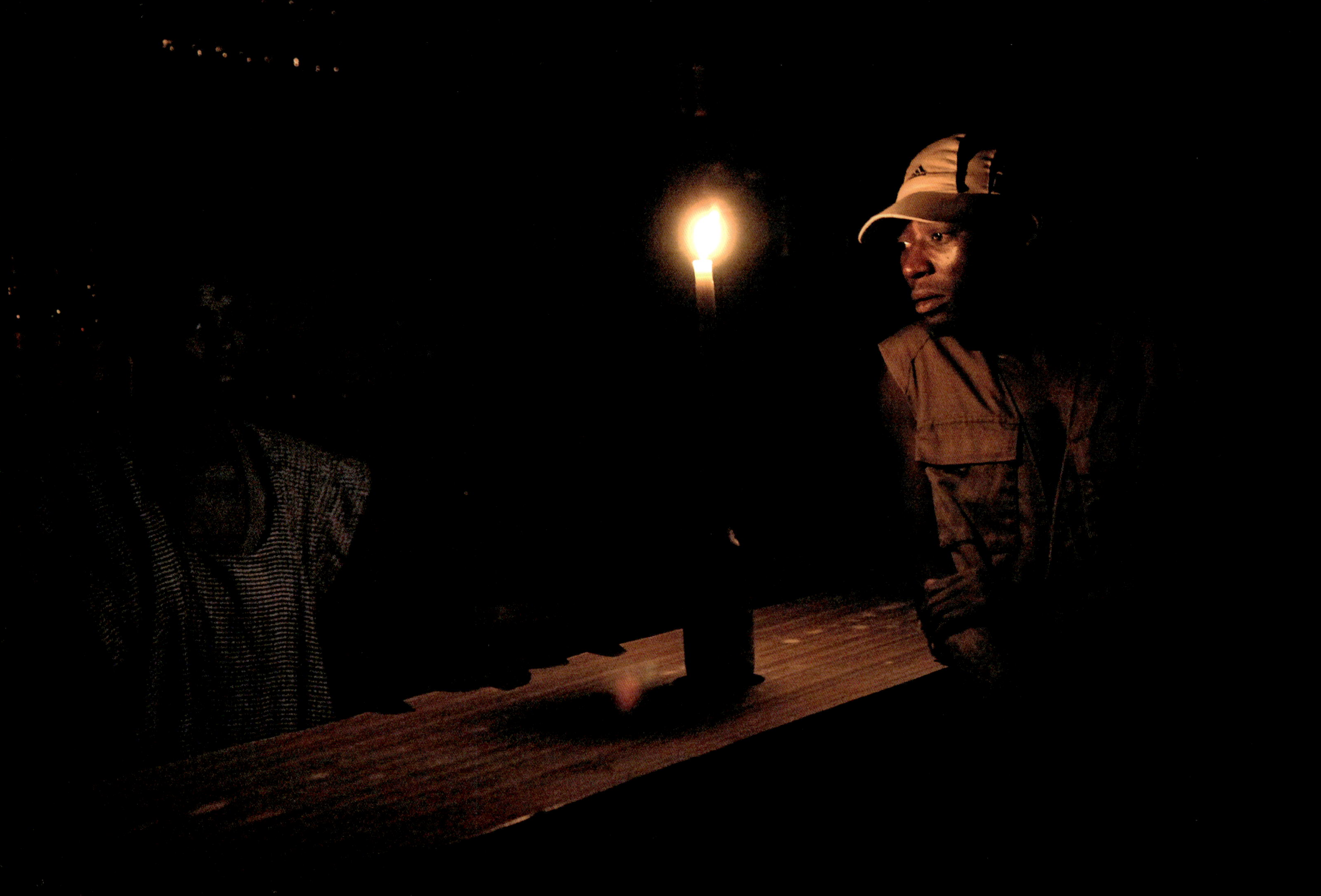

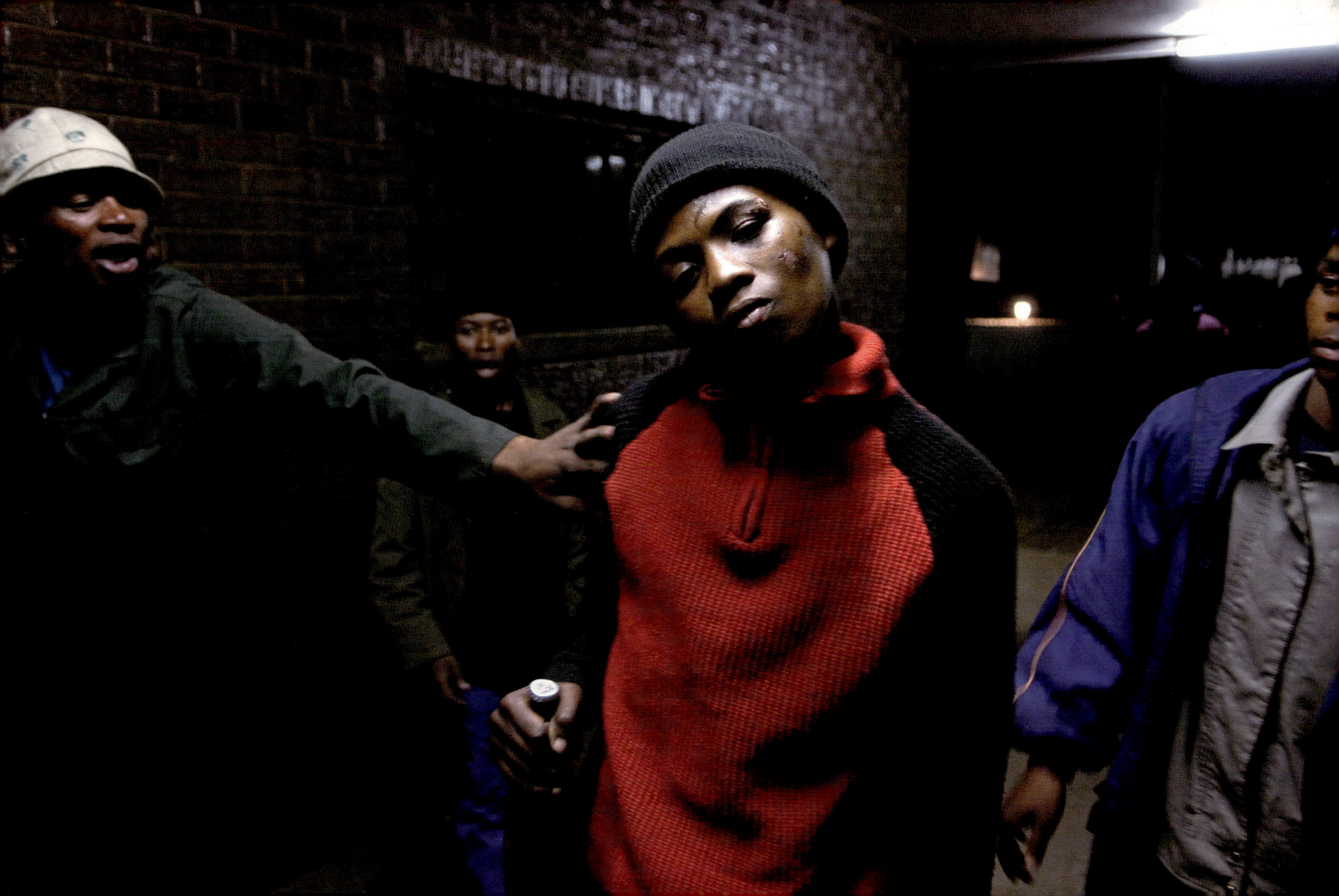

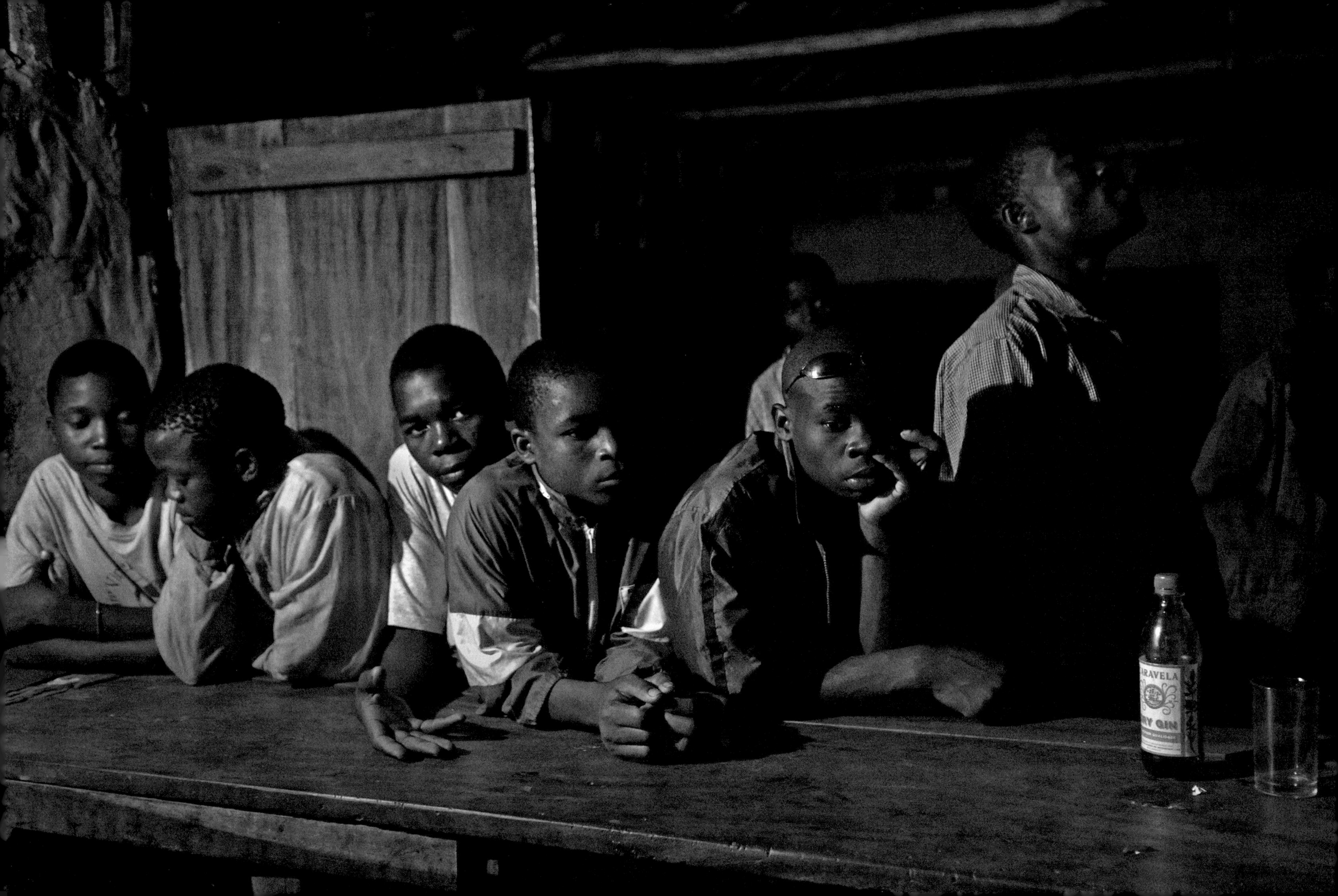

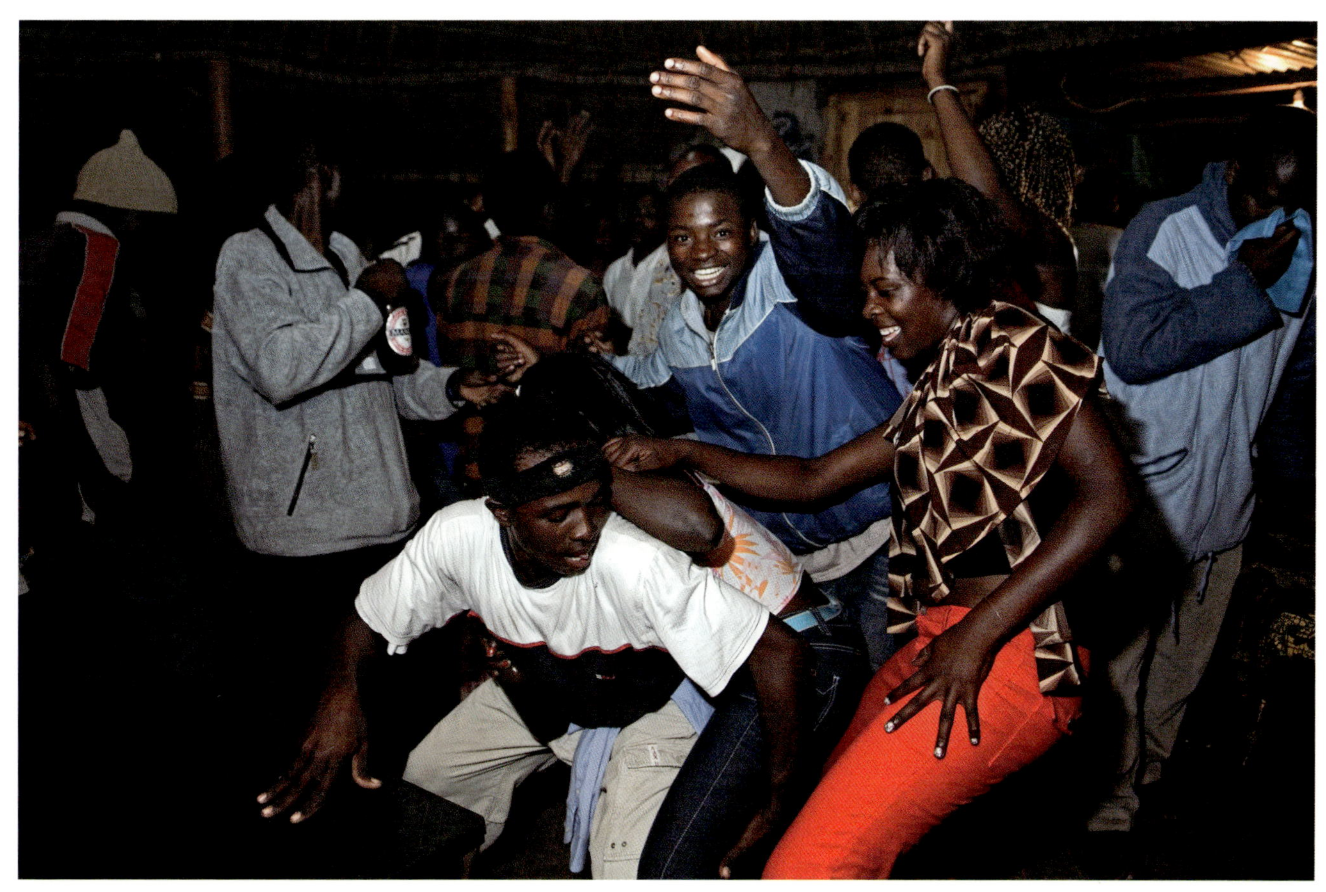

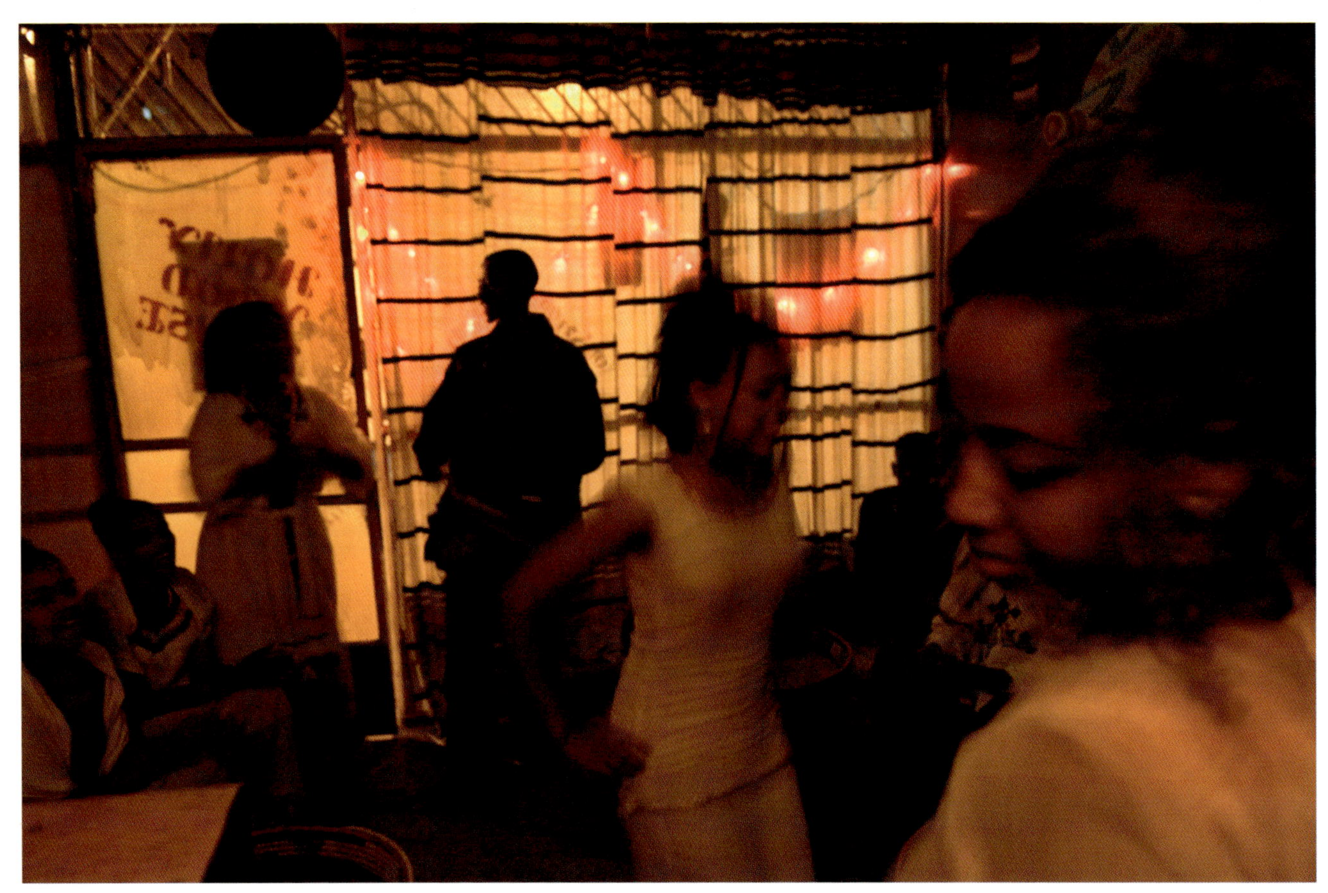

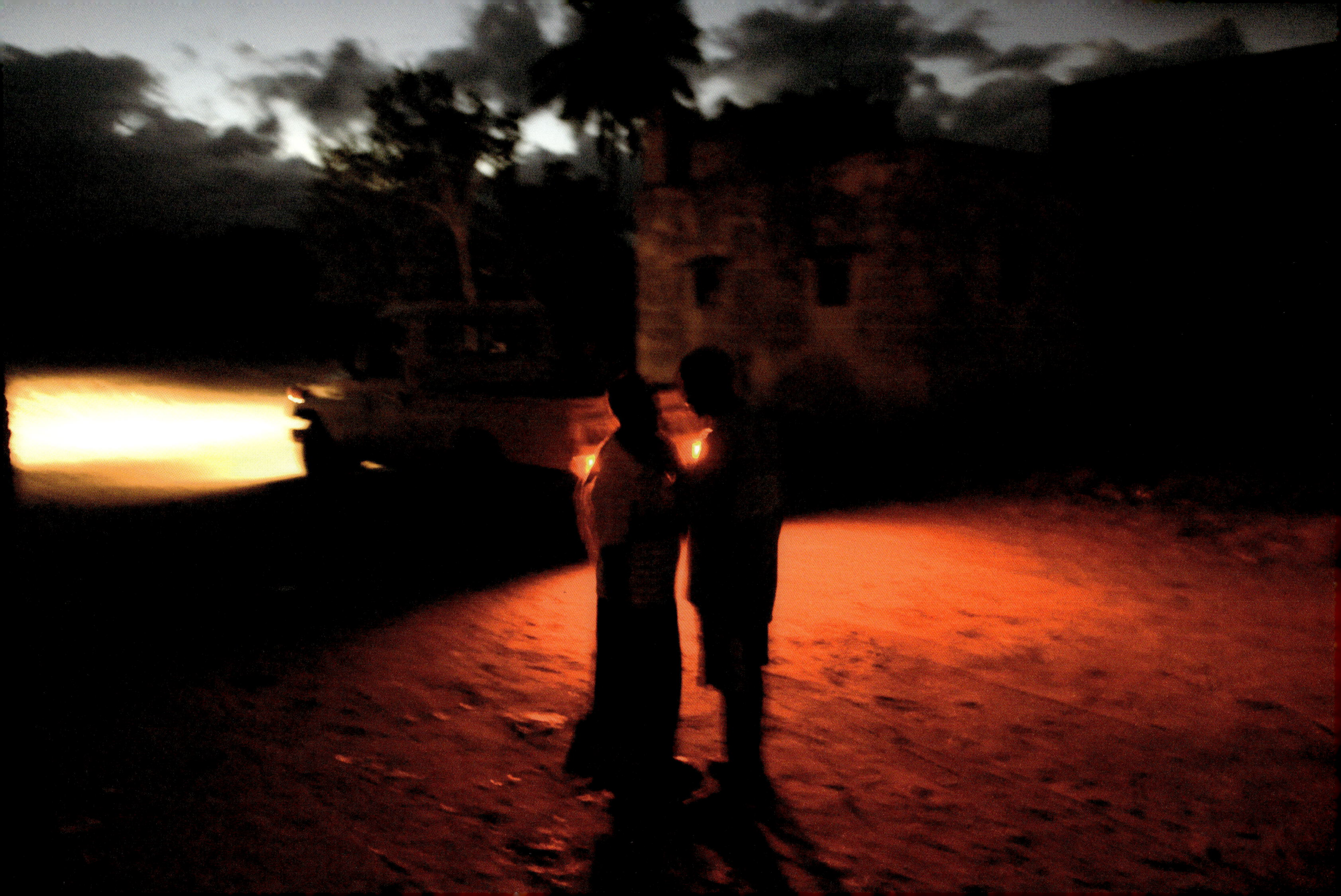

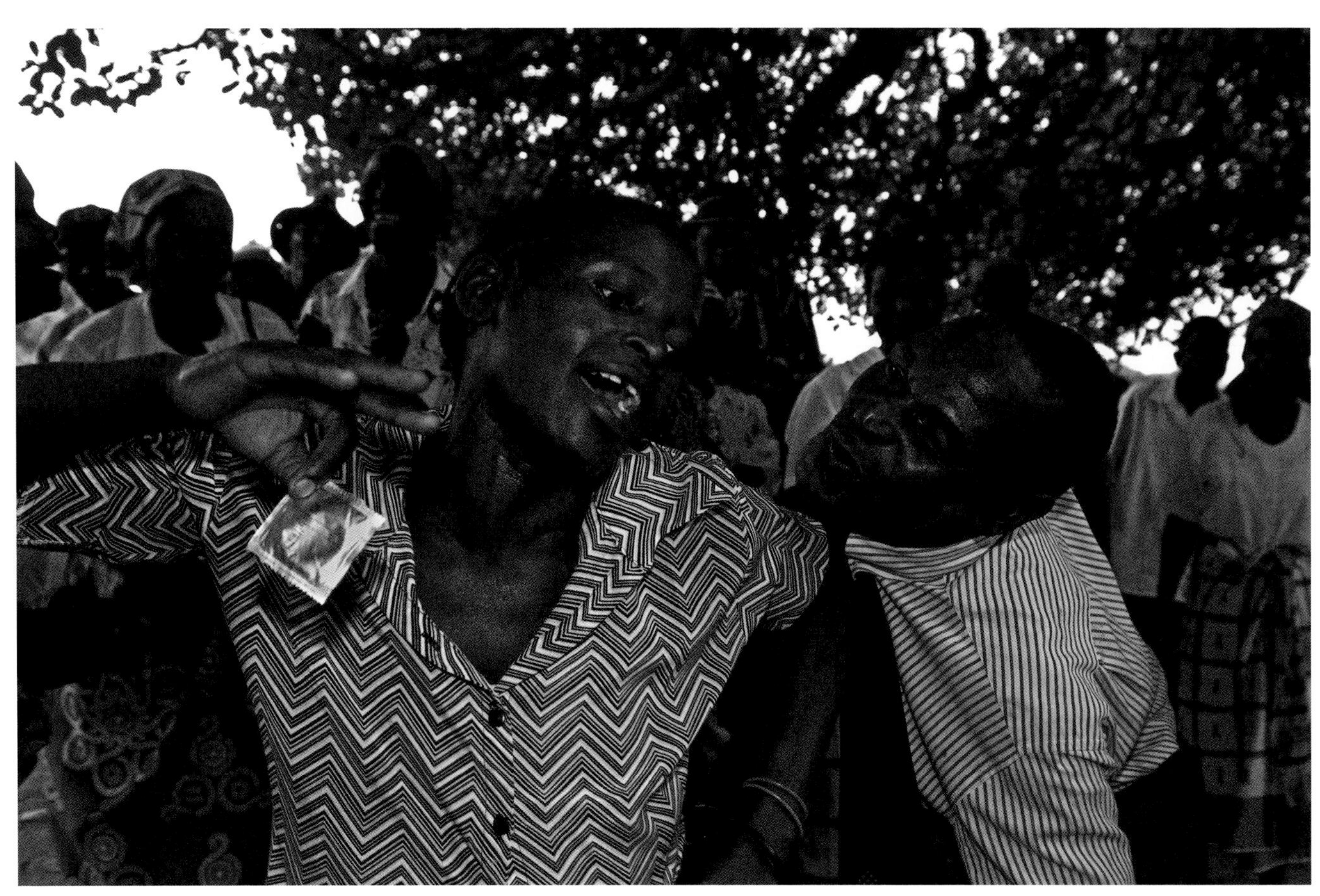

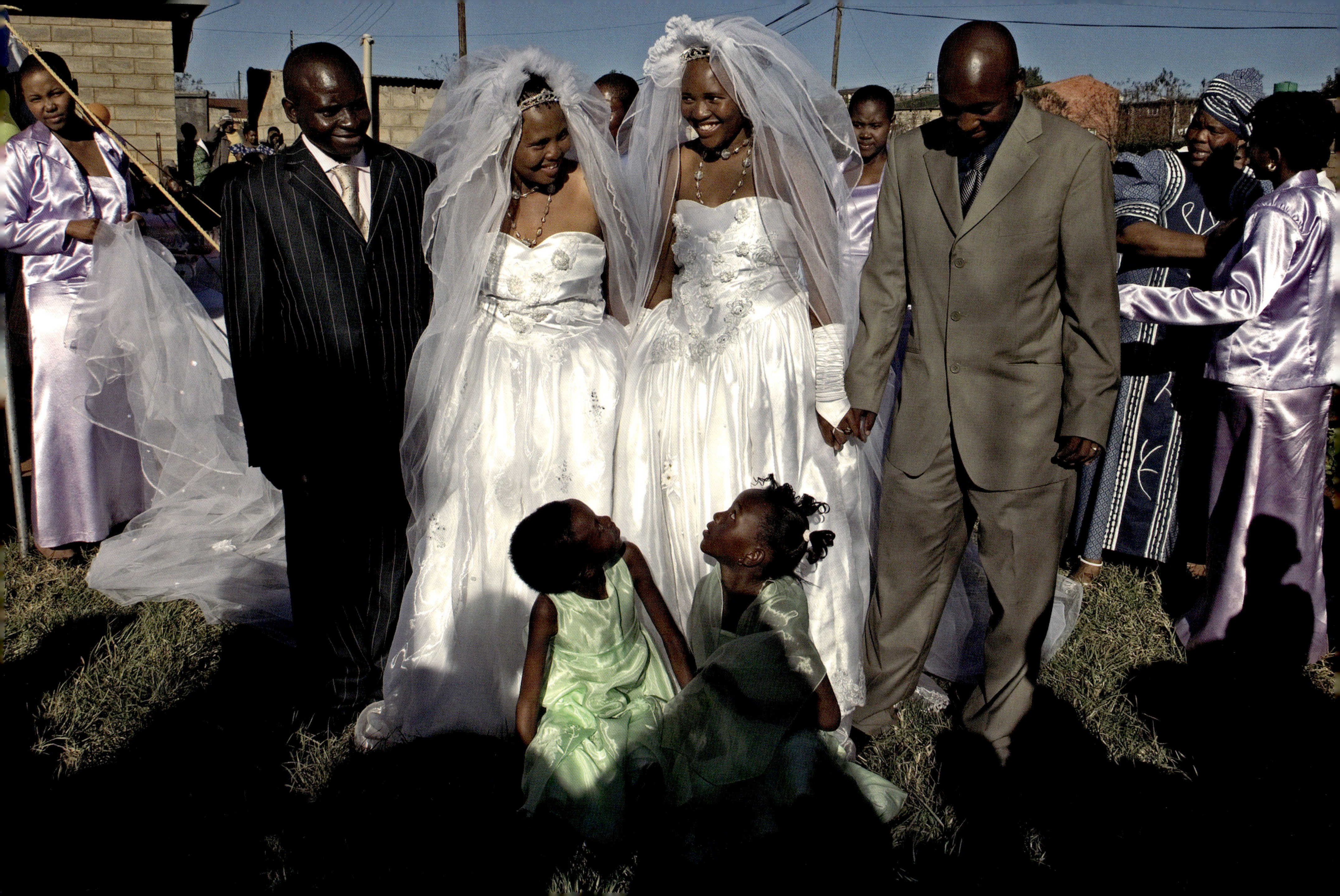

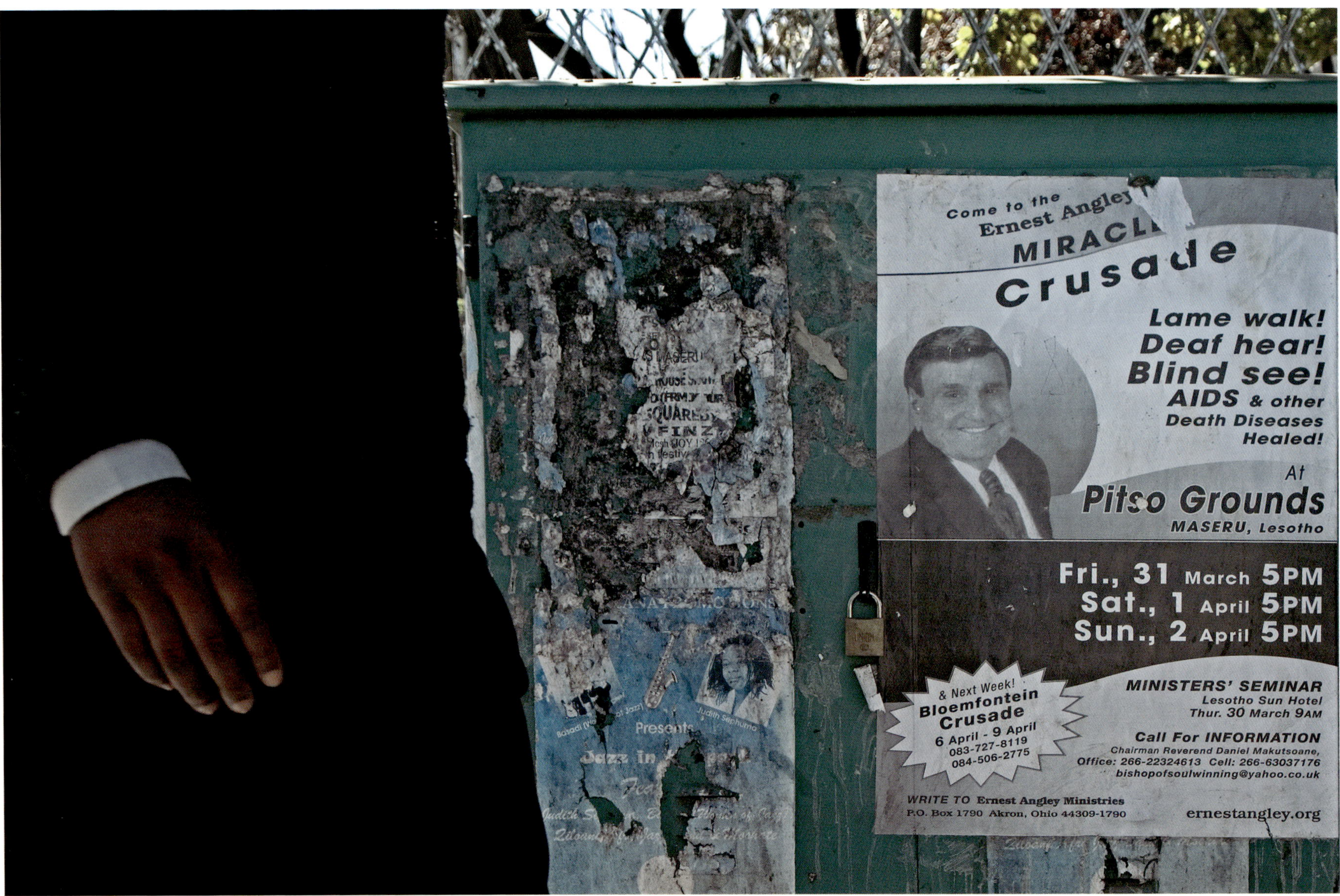

Come to the
Ernest Angley
MIRACLE
Crusade
Lame walk!
Deaf hear!
Blind see!
AIDS & other
Death Diseases
Healed!
At
Pitso Grounds
MASERU, Lesotho
Fri., 31 March 5PM
Sat., 1 April 5PM
Sun., 2 April 5PM
& Next Week!
Bloemfontein
Crusade
6 April - 9 April
083-727-8119
084-506-2775
MINISTERS' SEMINAR
Lesotho Sun Hotel
Thur. 30 March 9AM
Call For INFORMATION
Chairman Reverend Daniel Makutsoane,
Office: 266-22324613 Cell: 266-63037176
bishopofsoulwinning@yahoo.co.uk
WRITE TO Ernest Angley Ministries
P.O. Box 1790 Akron, Ohio 44309-1790
ernestangley.org

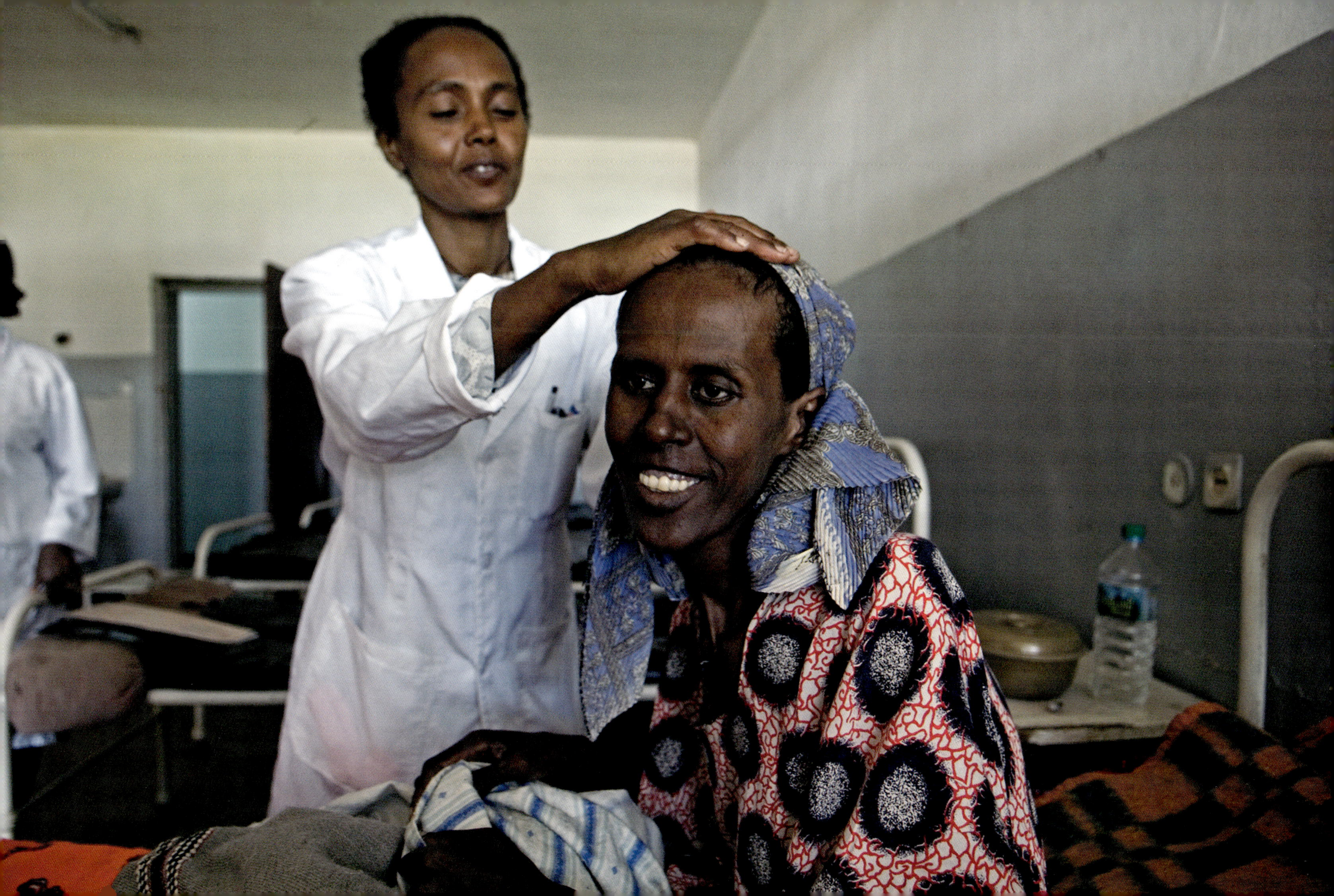

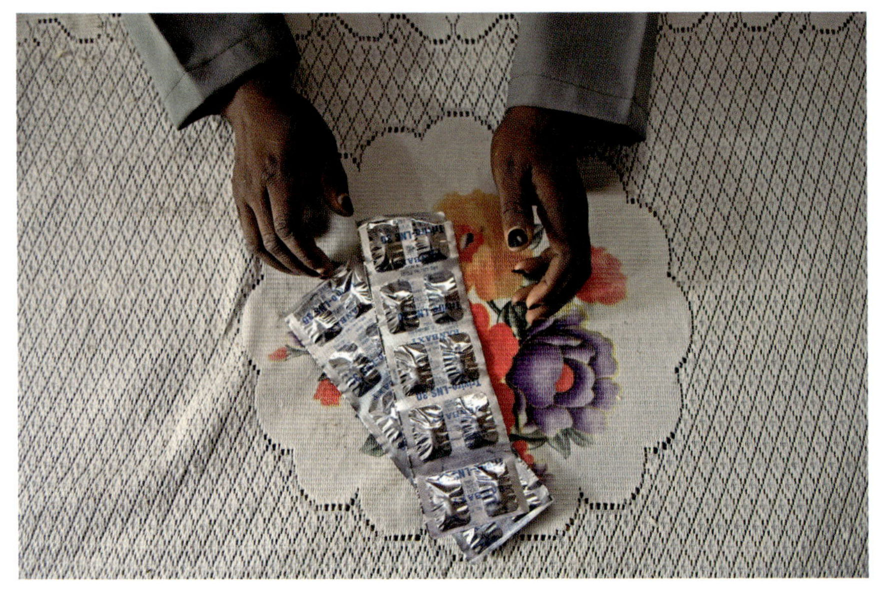
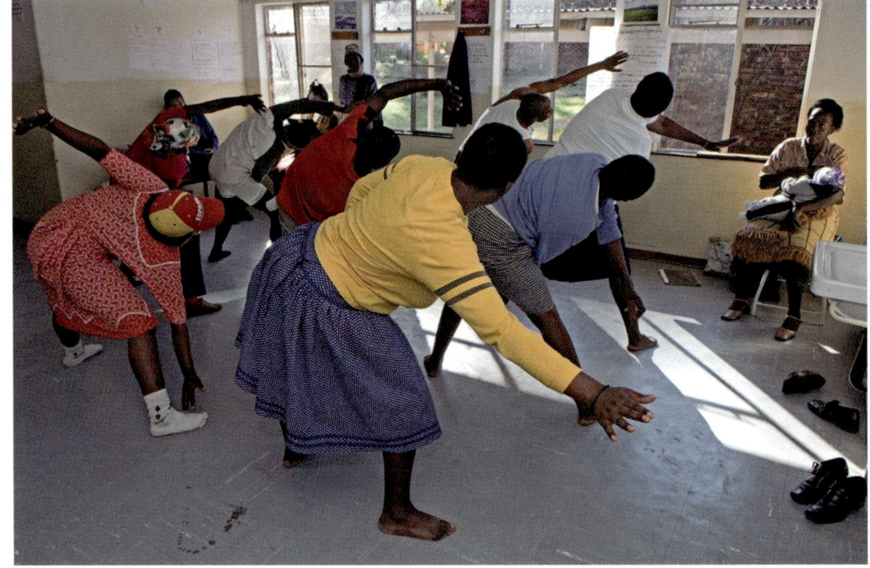

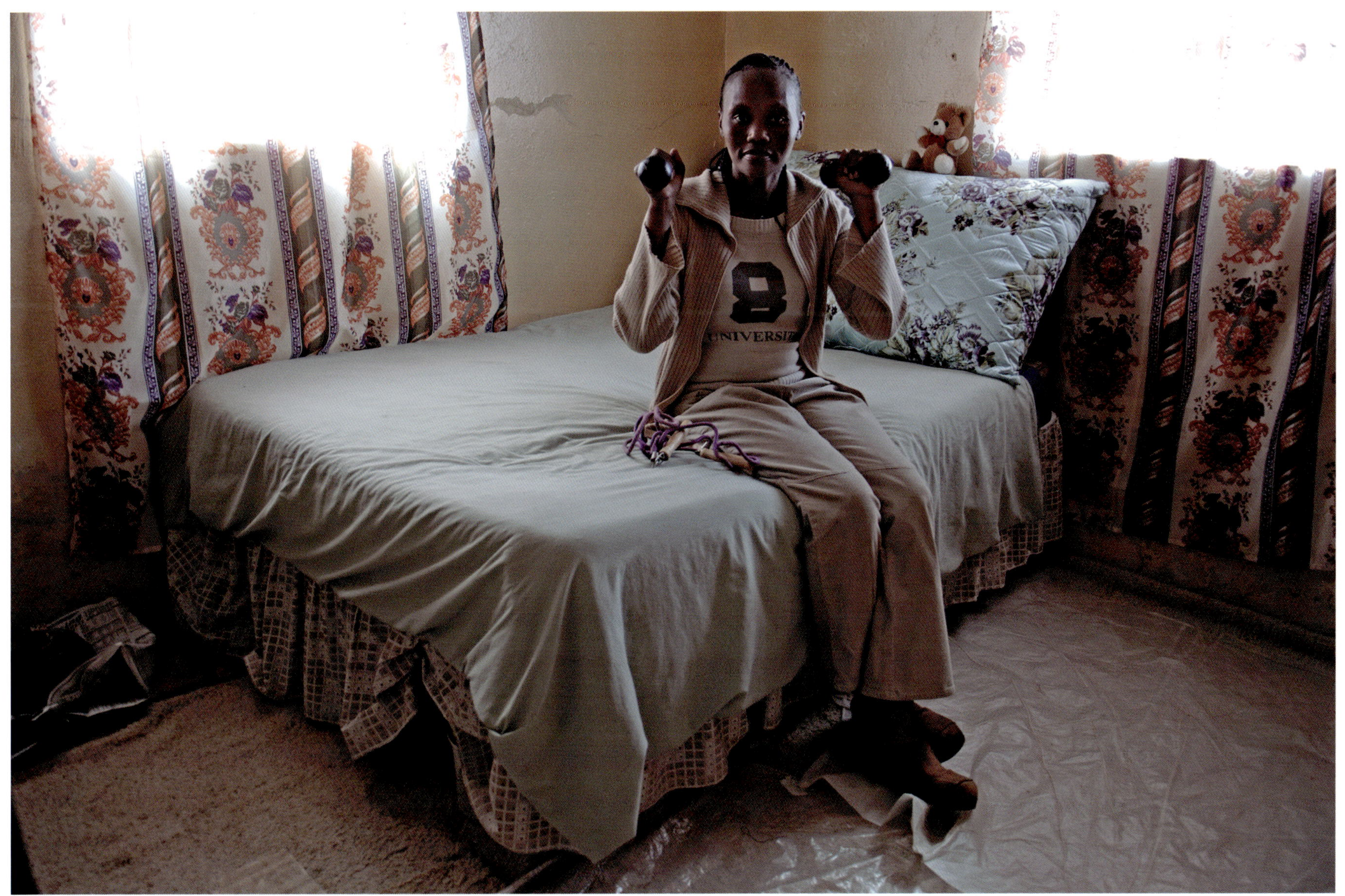

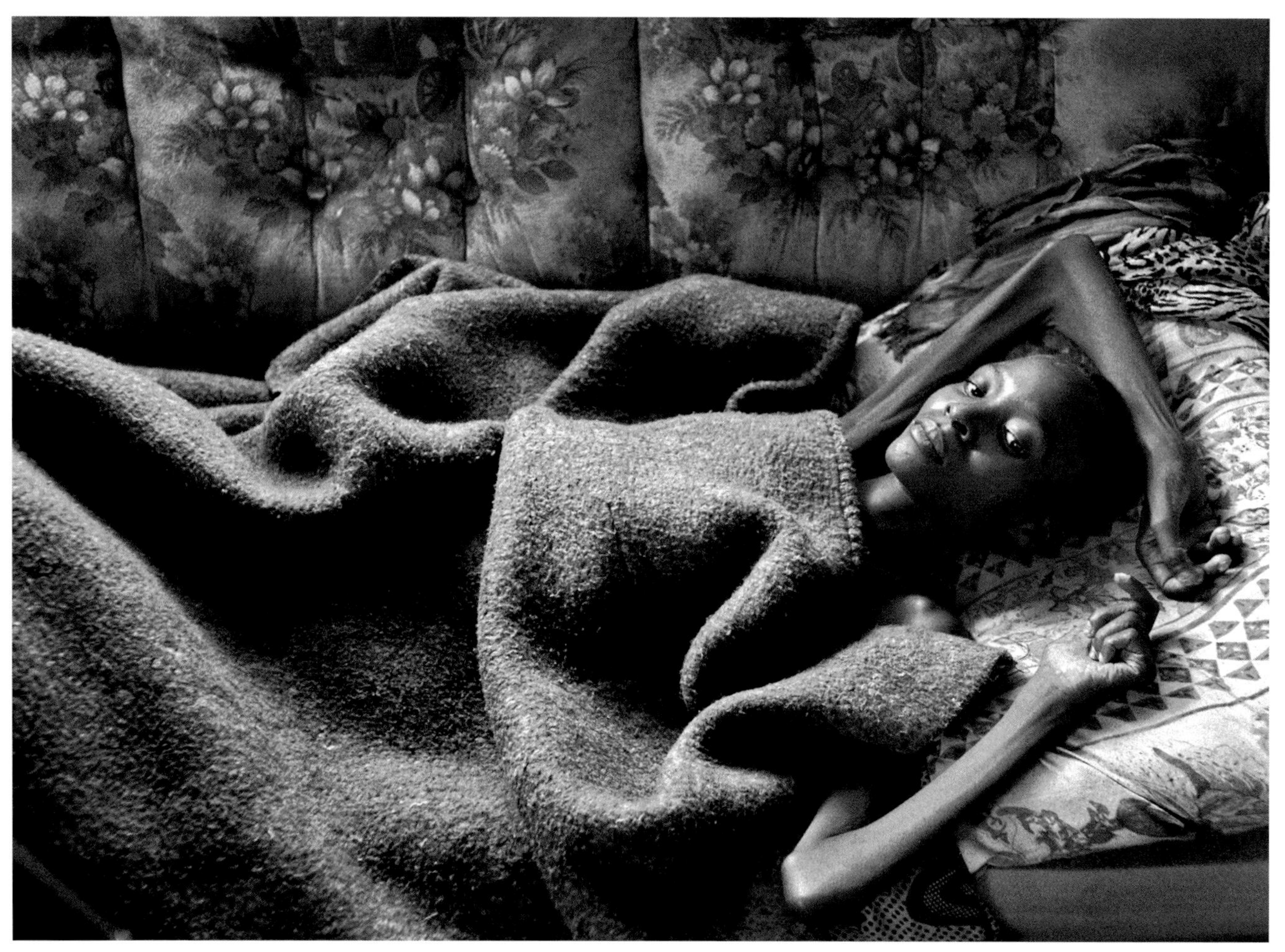

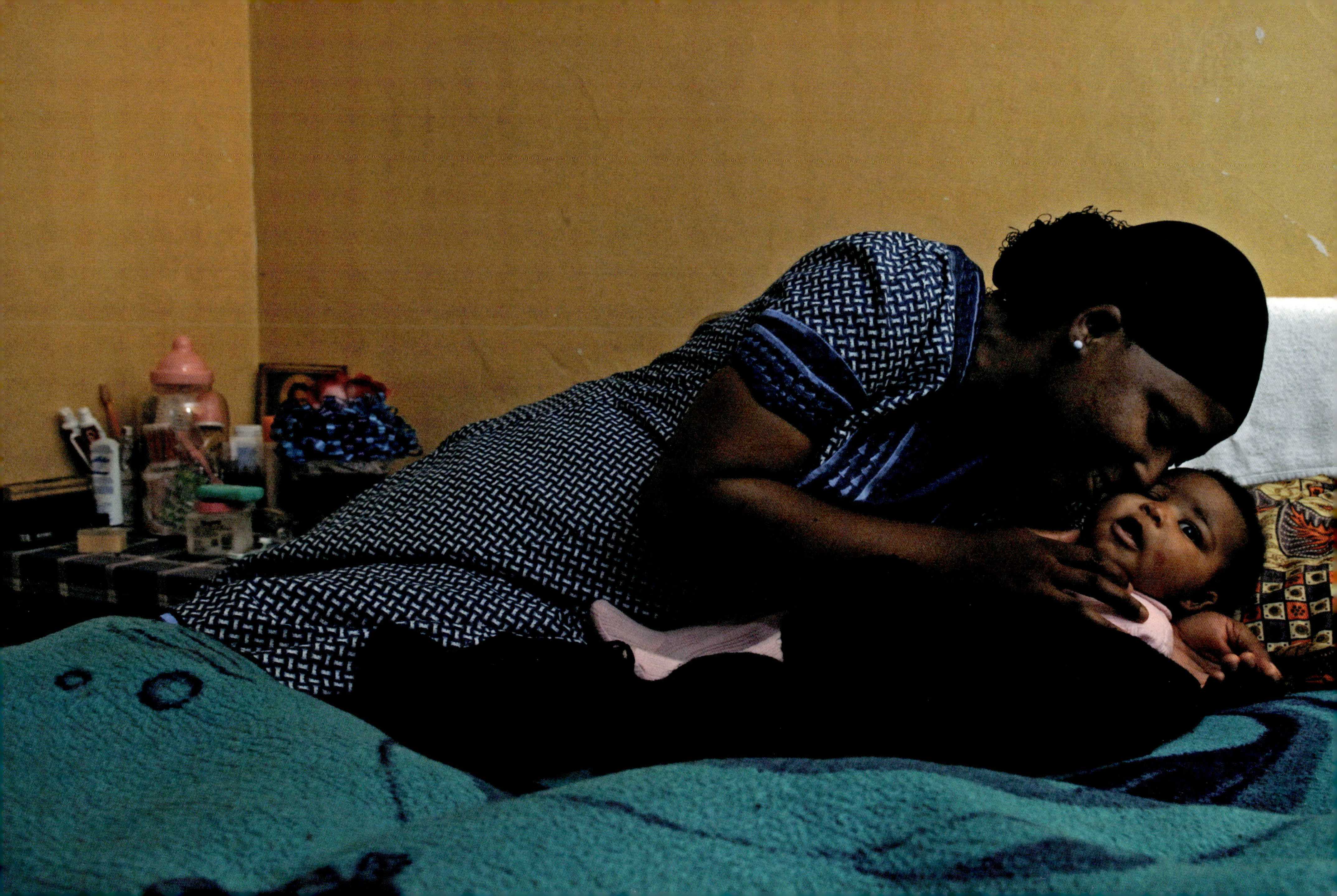

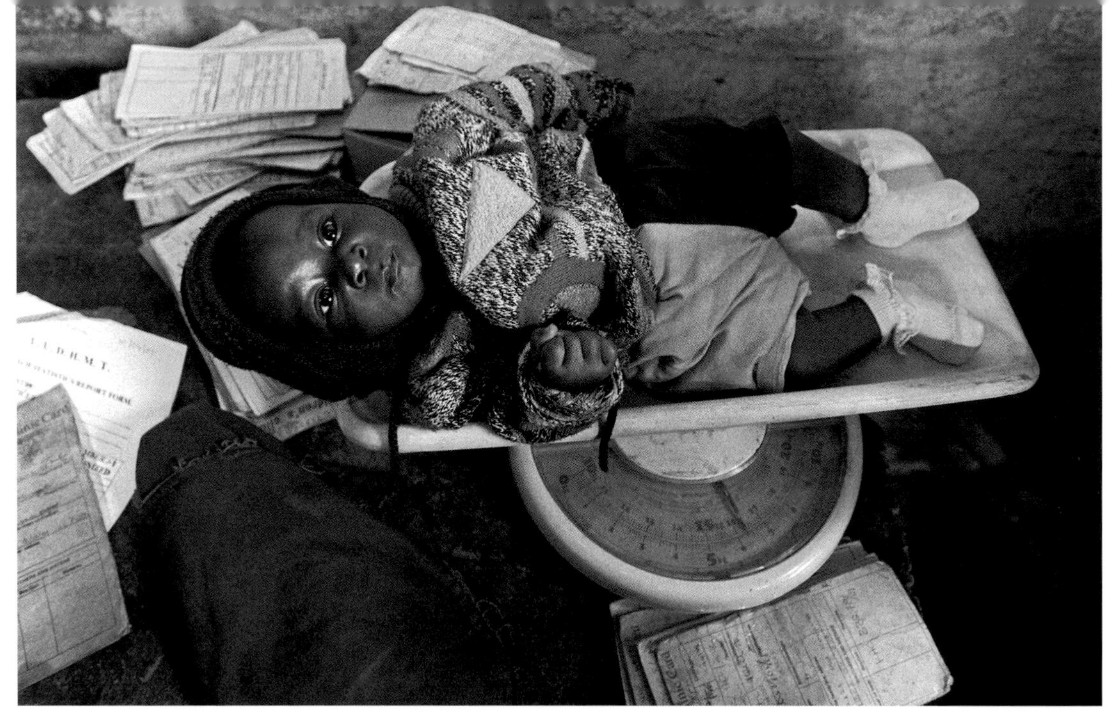

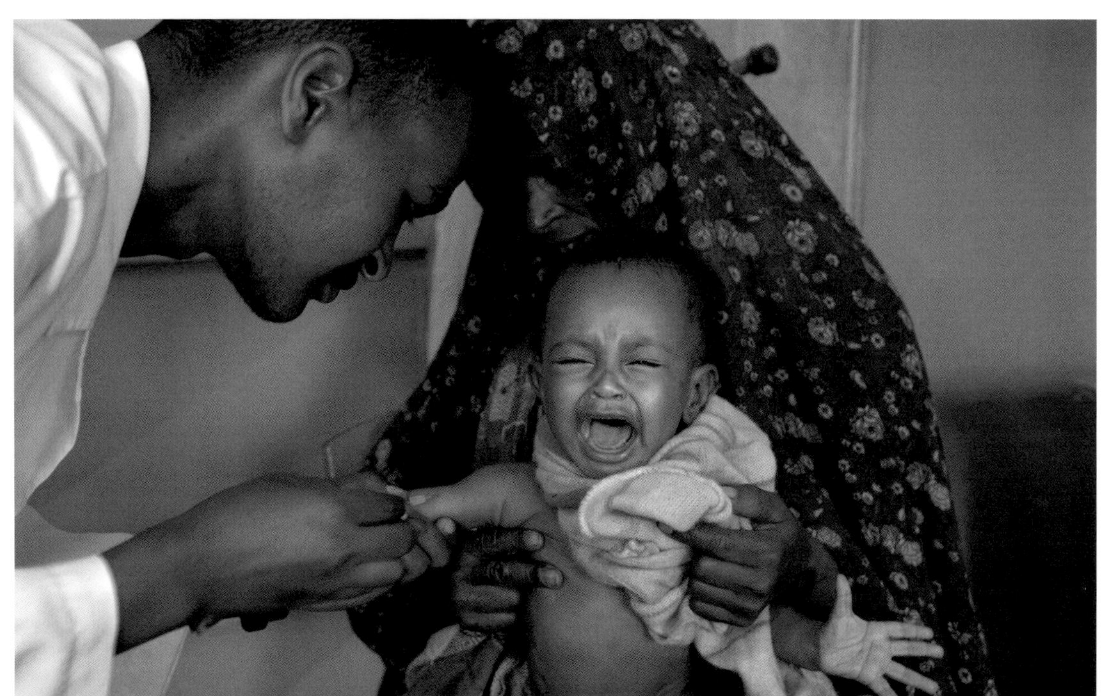

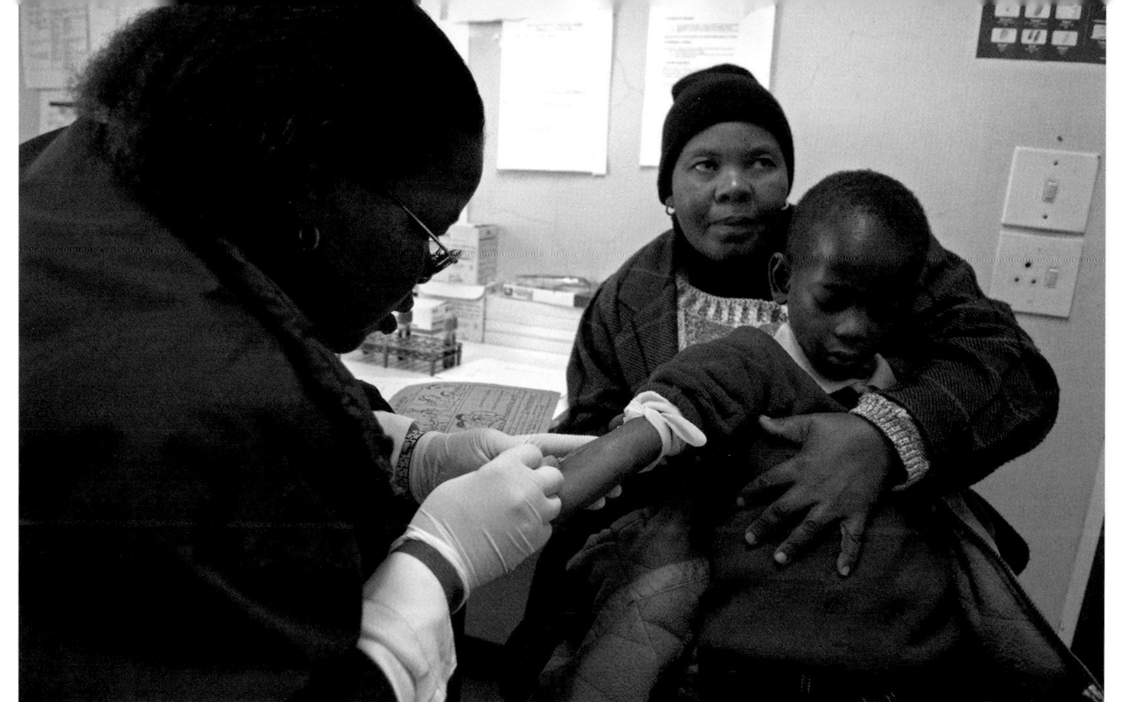

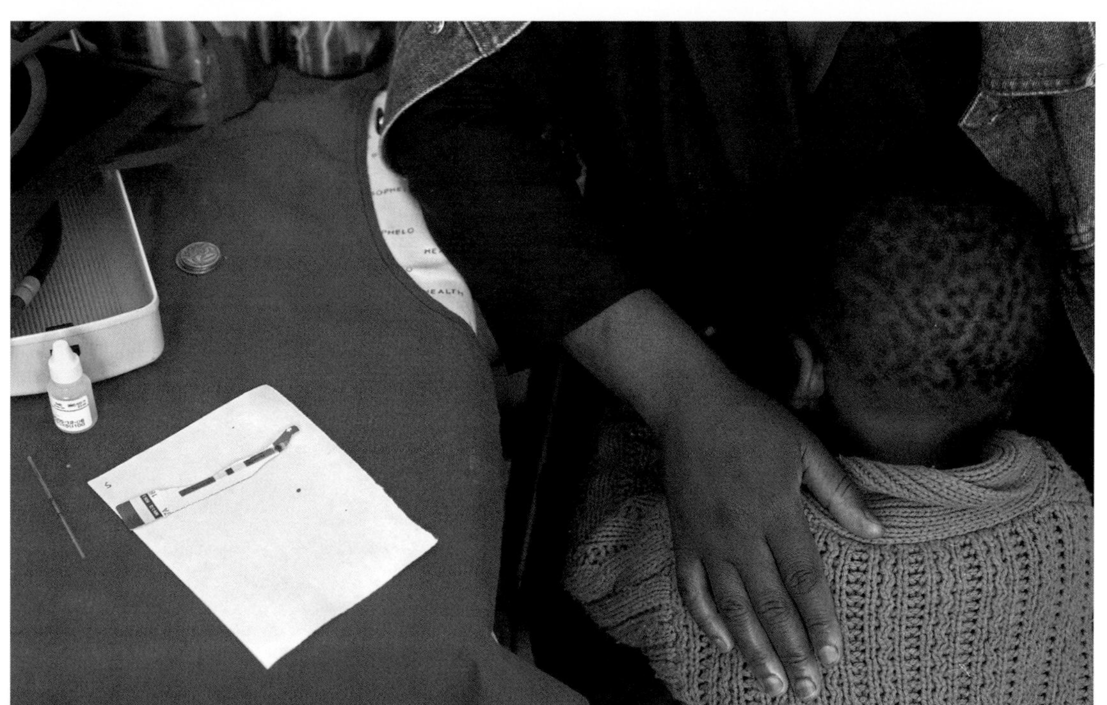

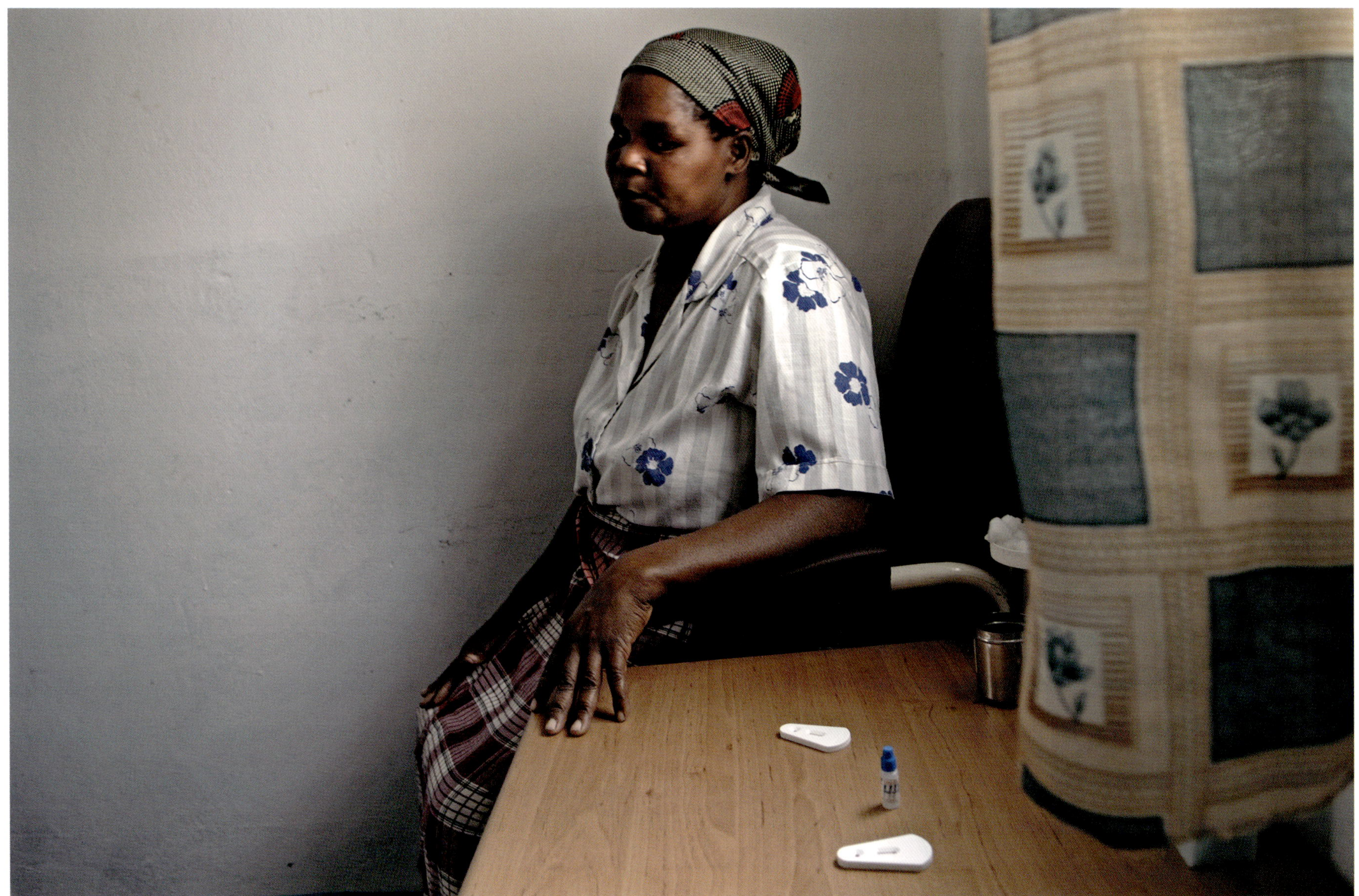

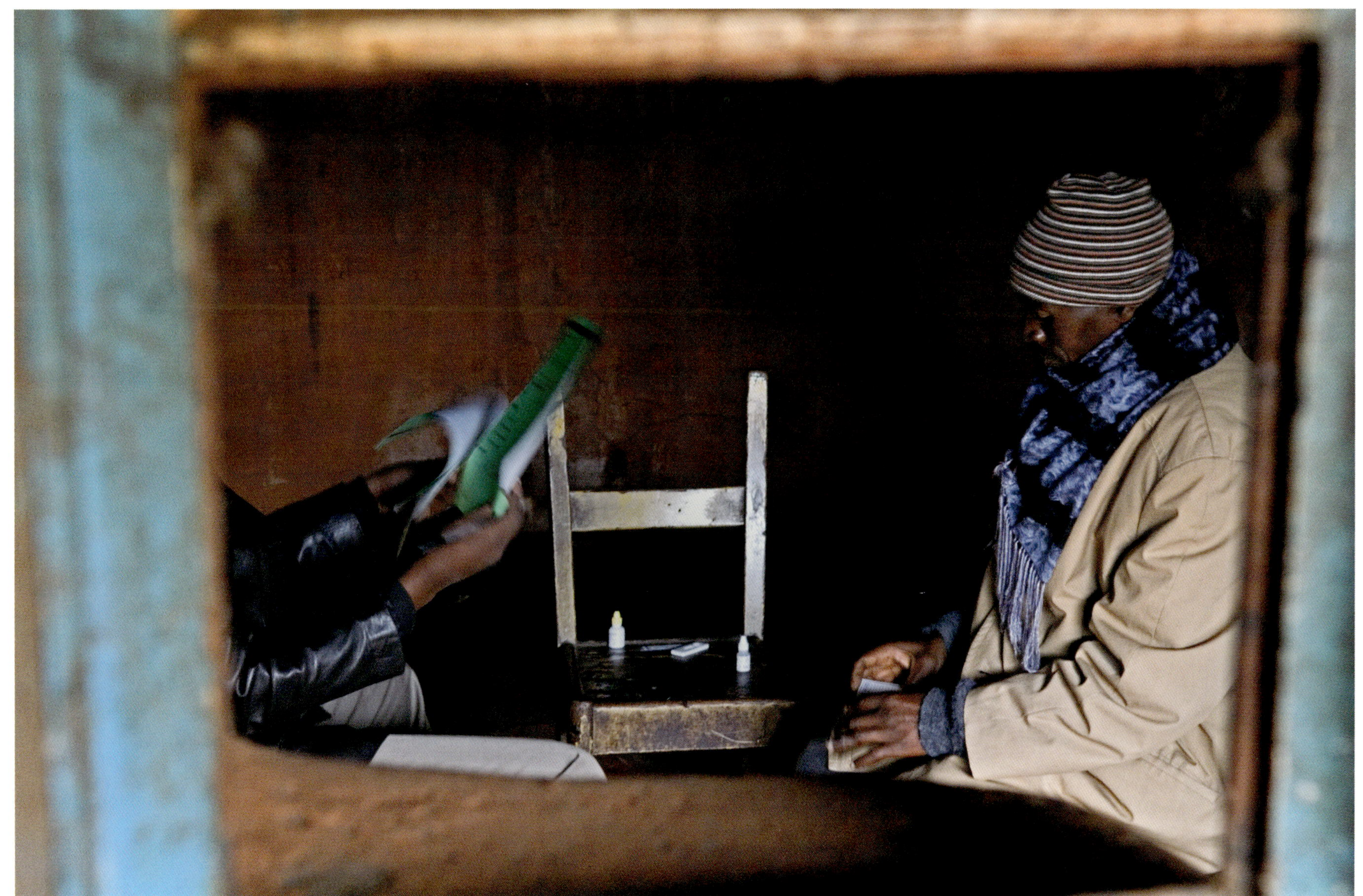

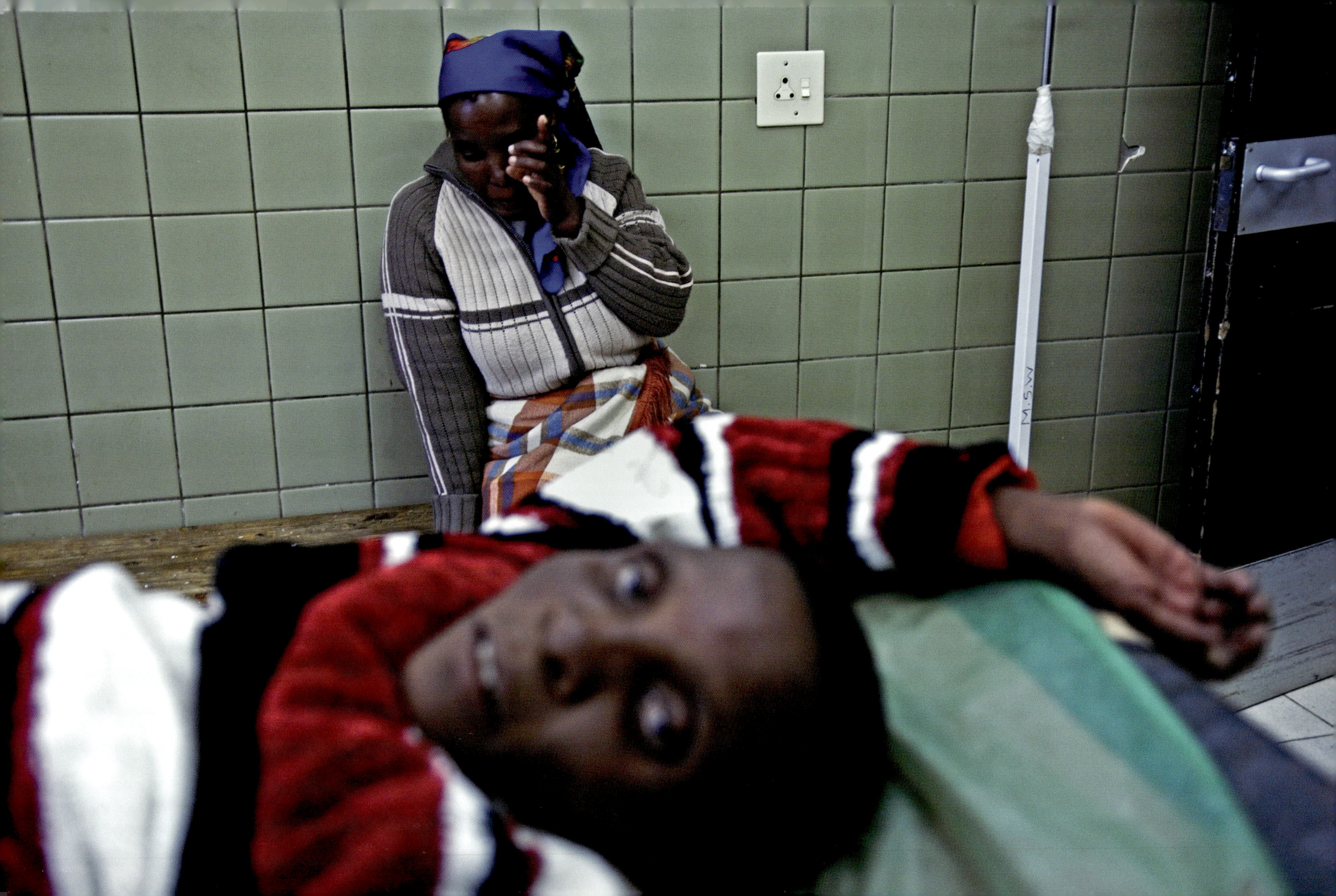

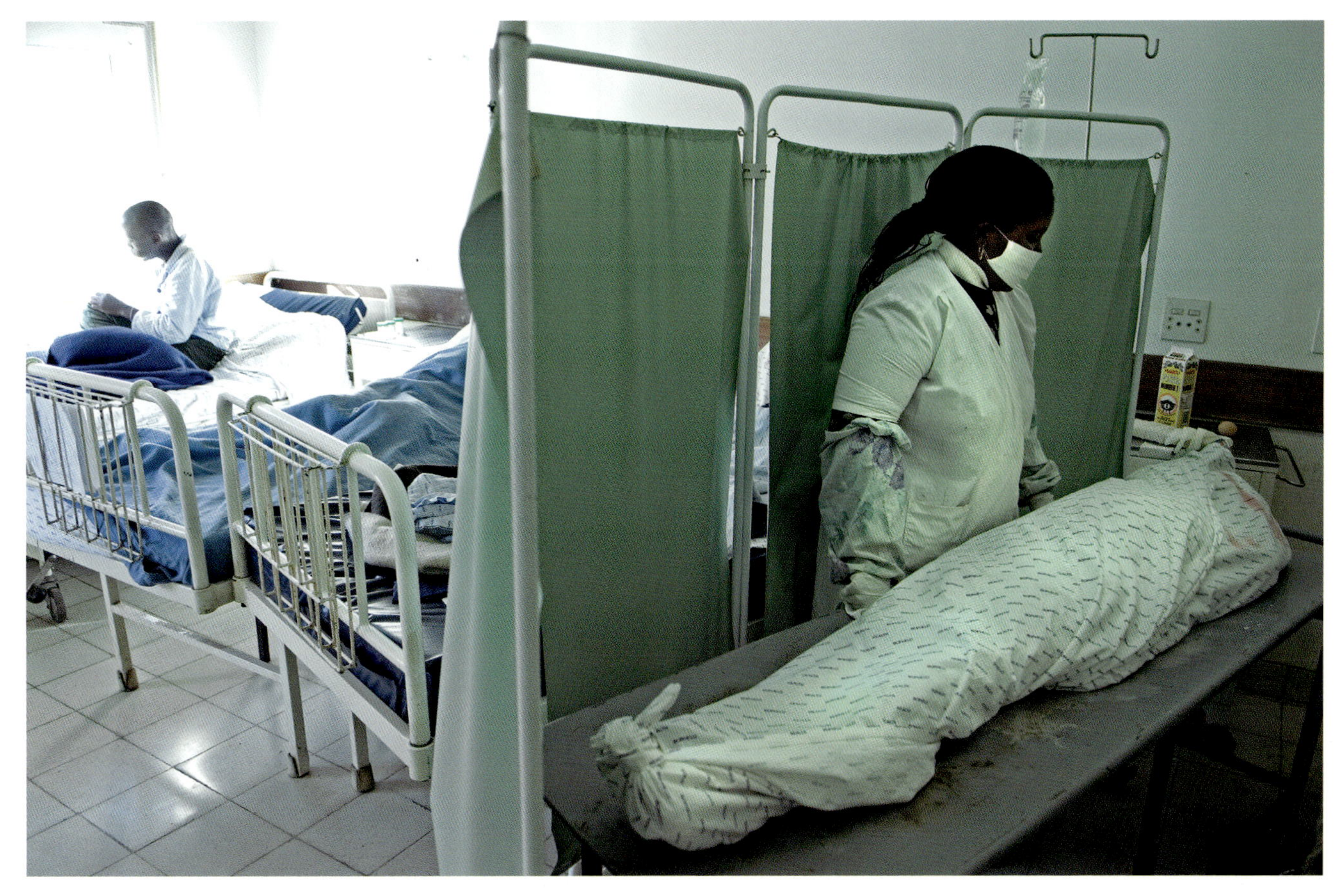

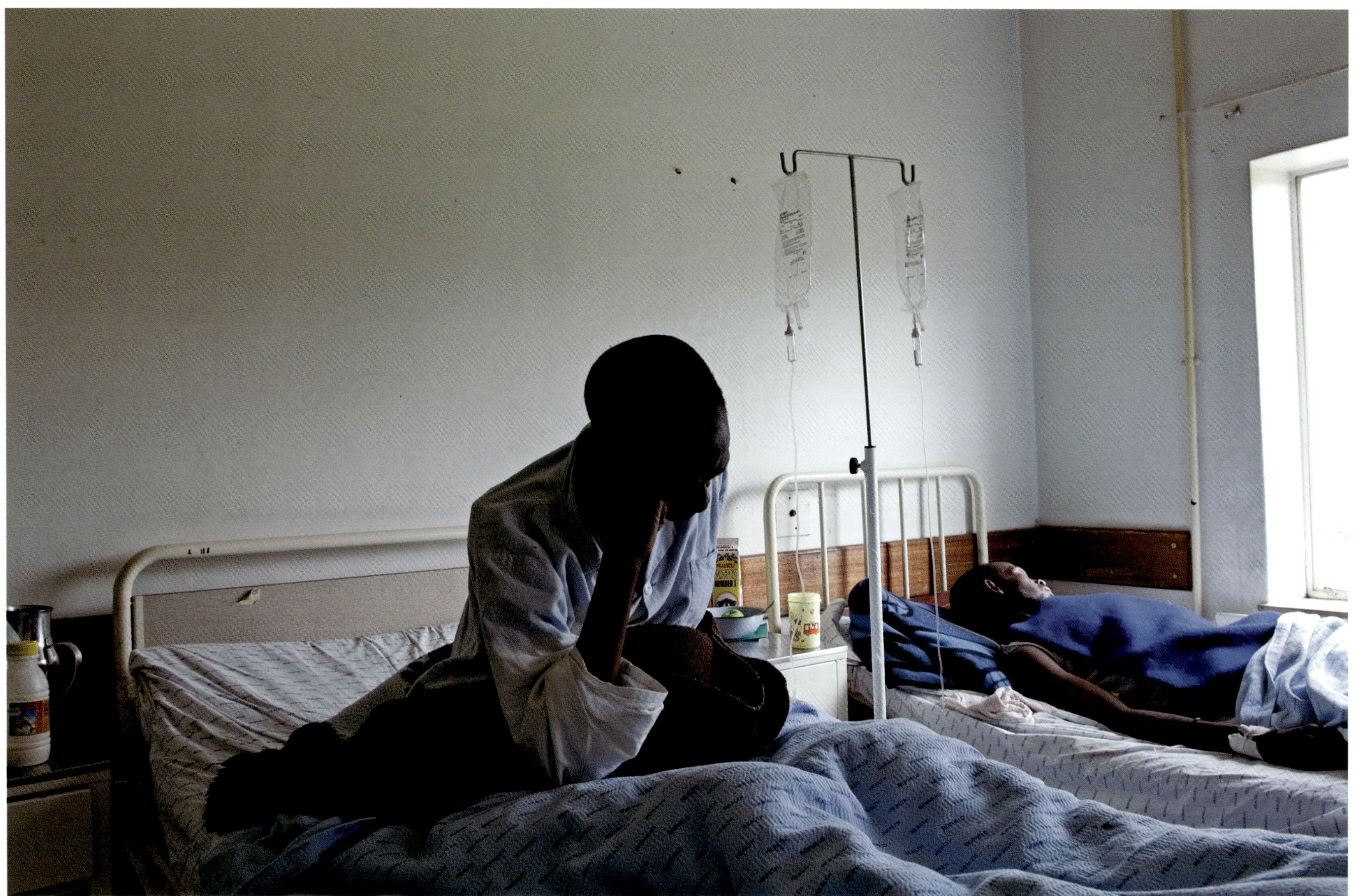

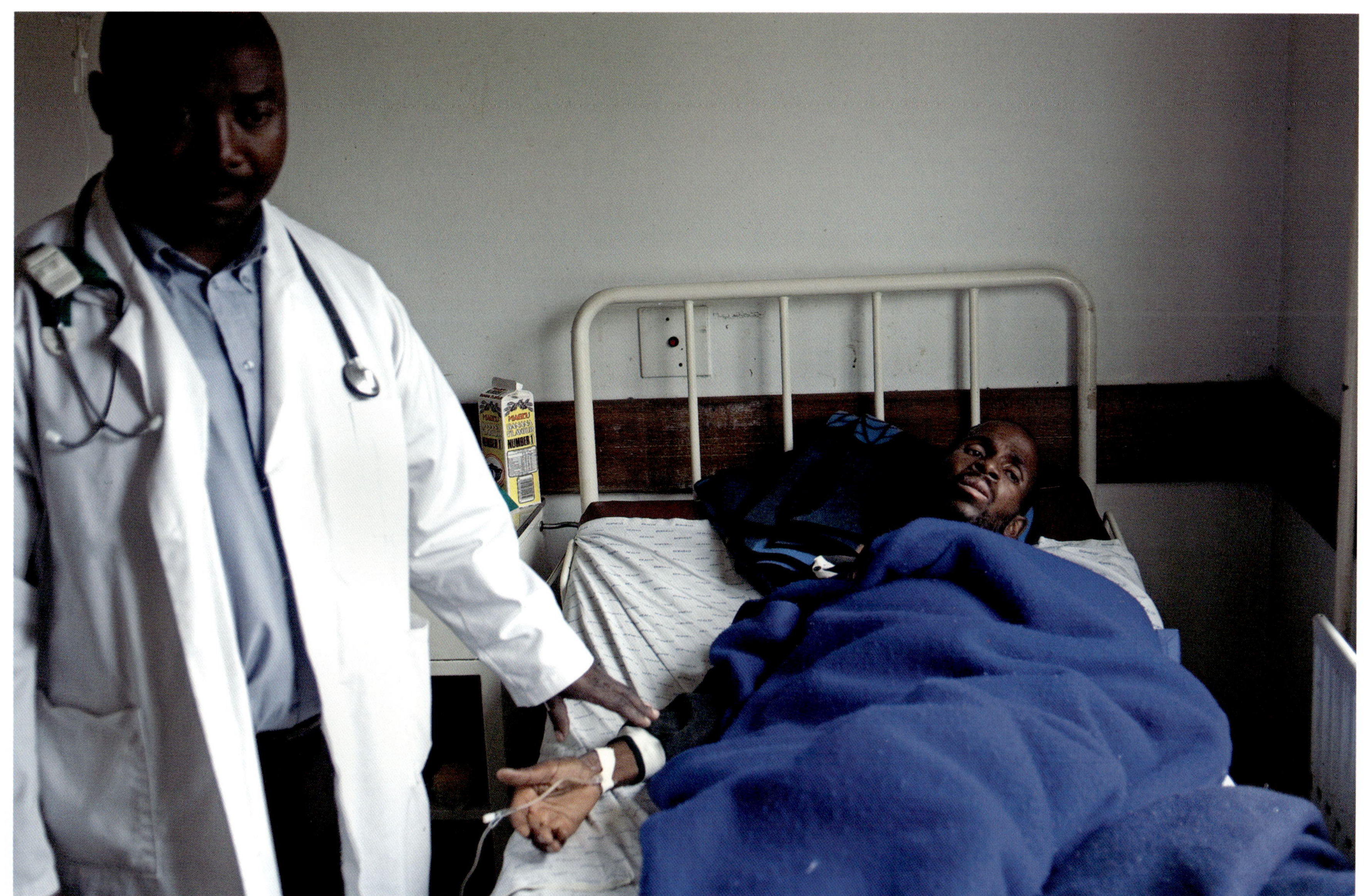

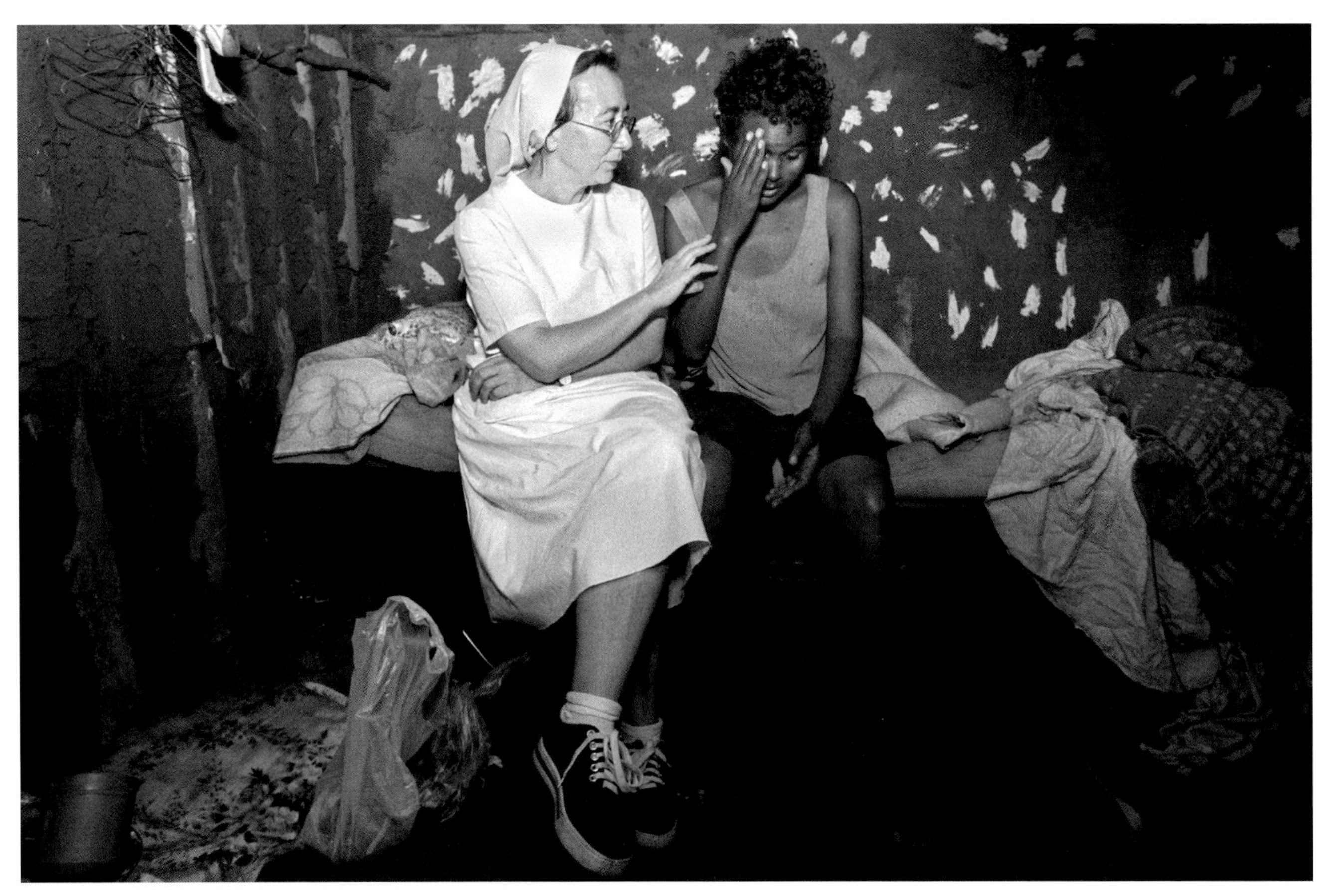

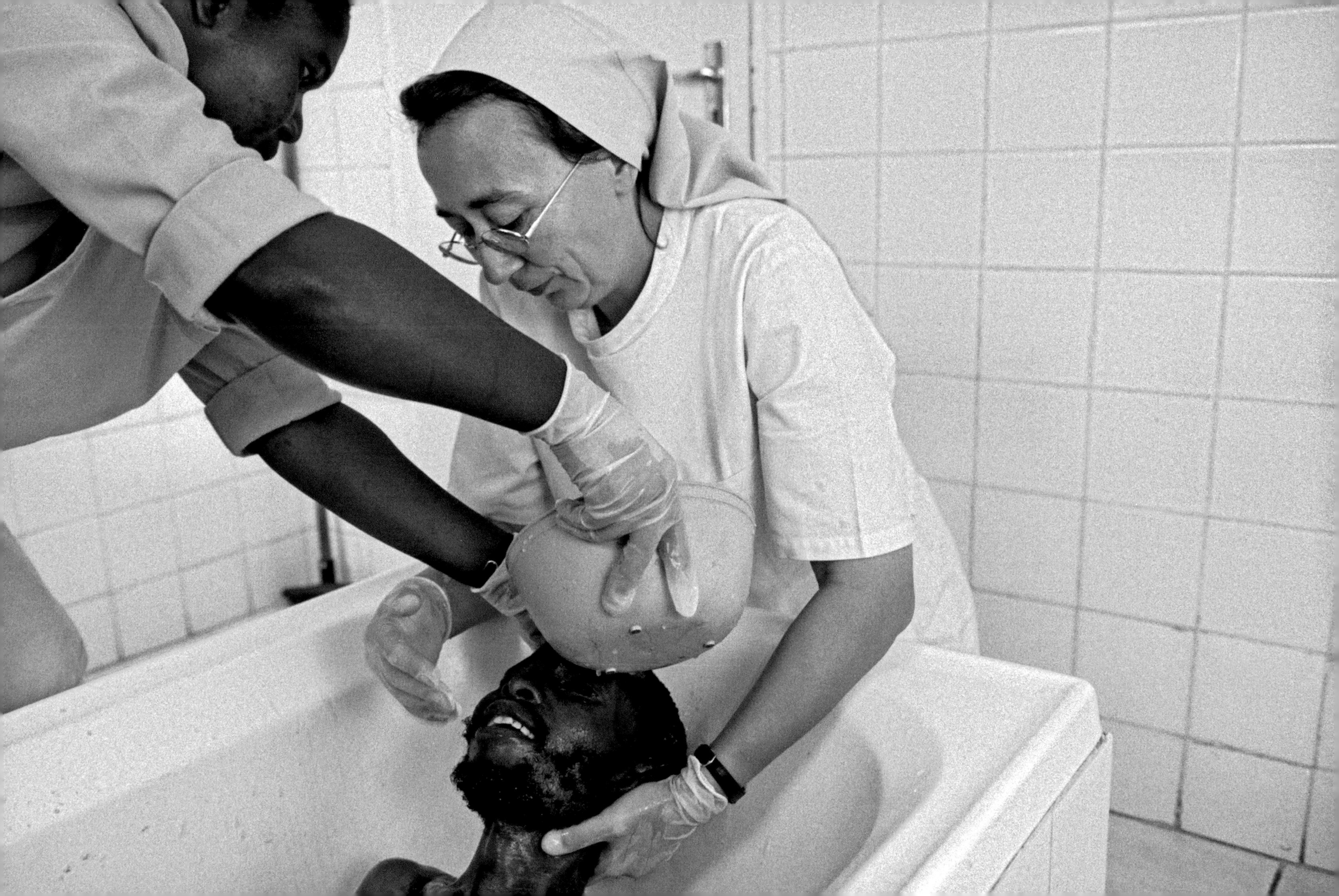

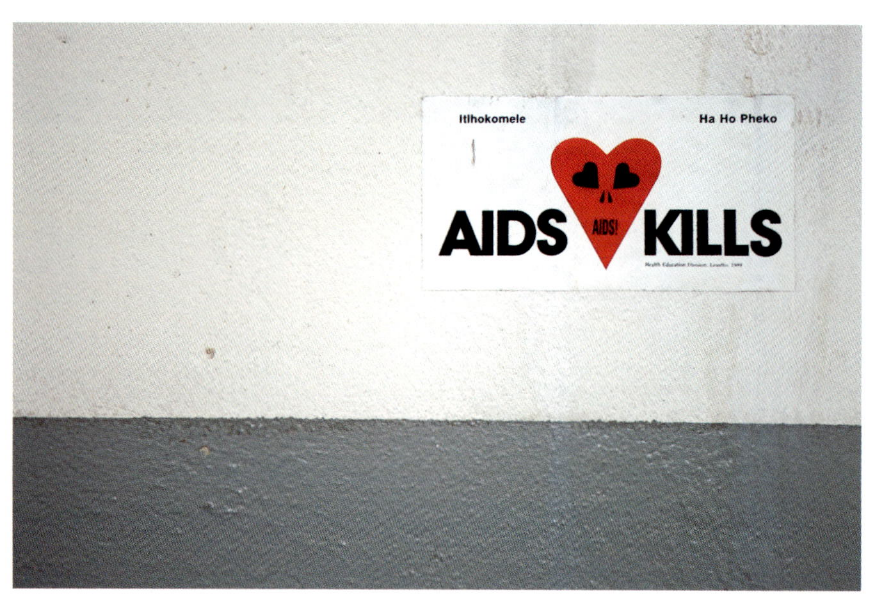
Itlhokomele
Ha Ho Pheko
AIDS
AIDS!
KILLS
Health Education Division, Lesotho, 1999

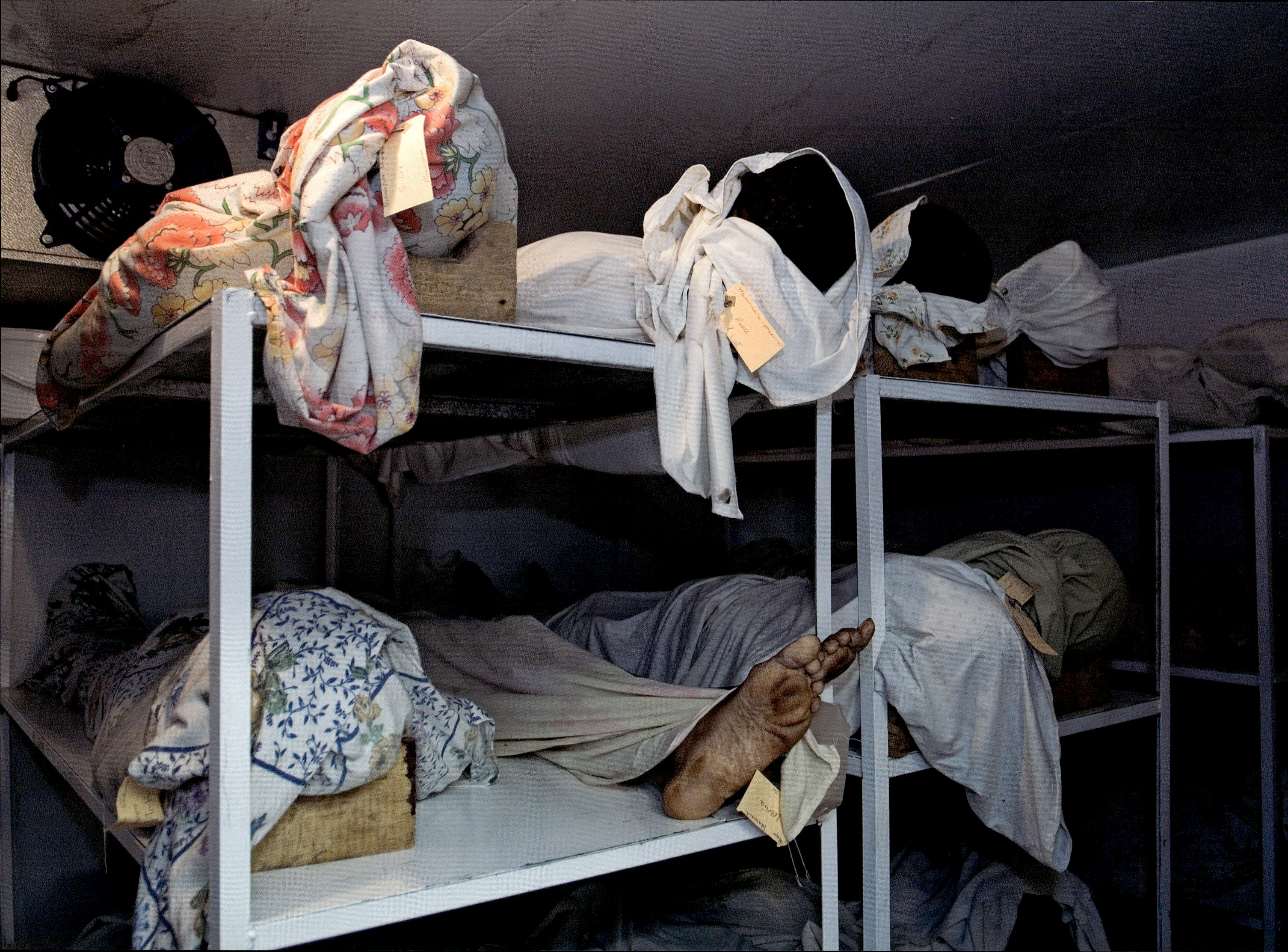

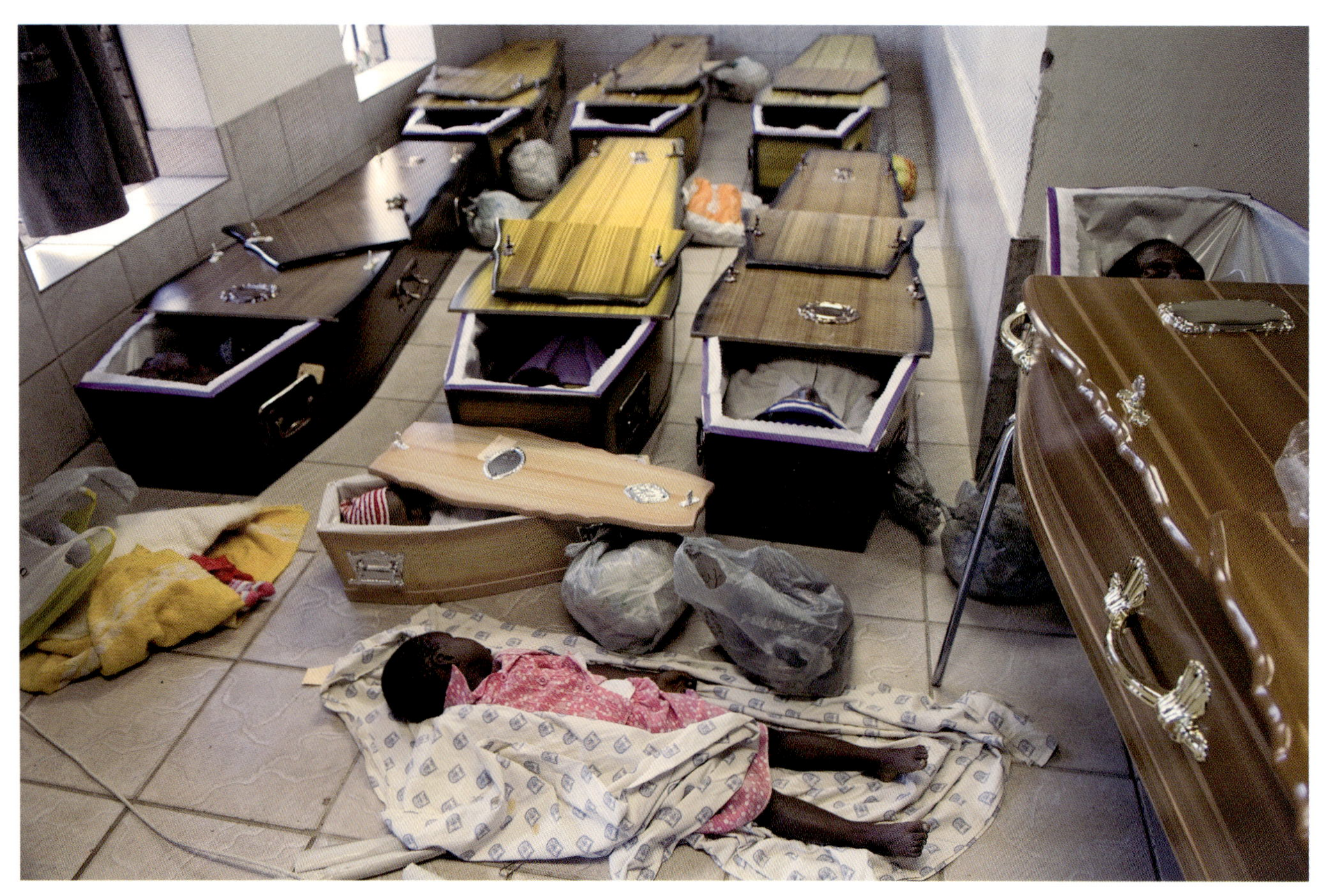

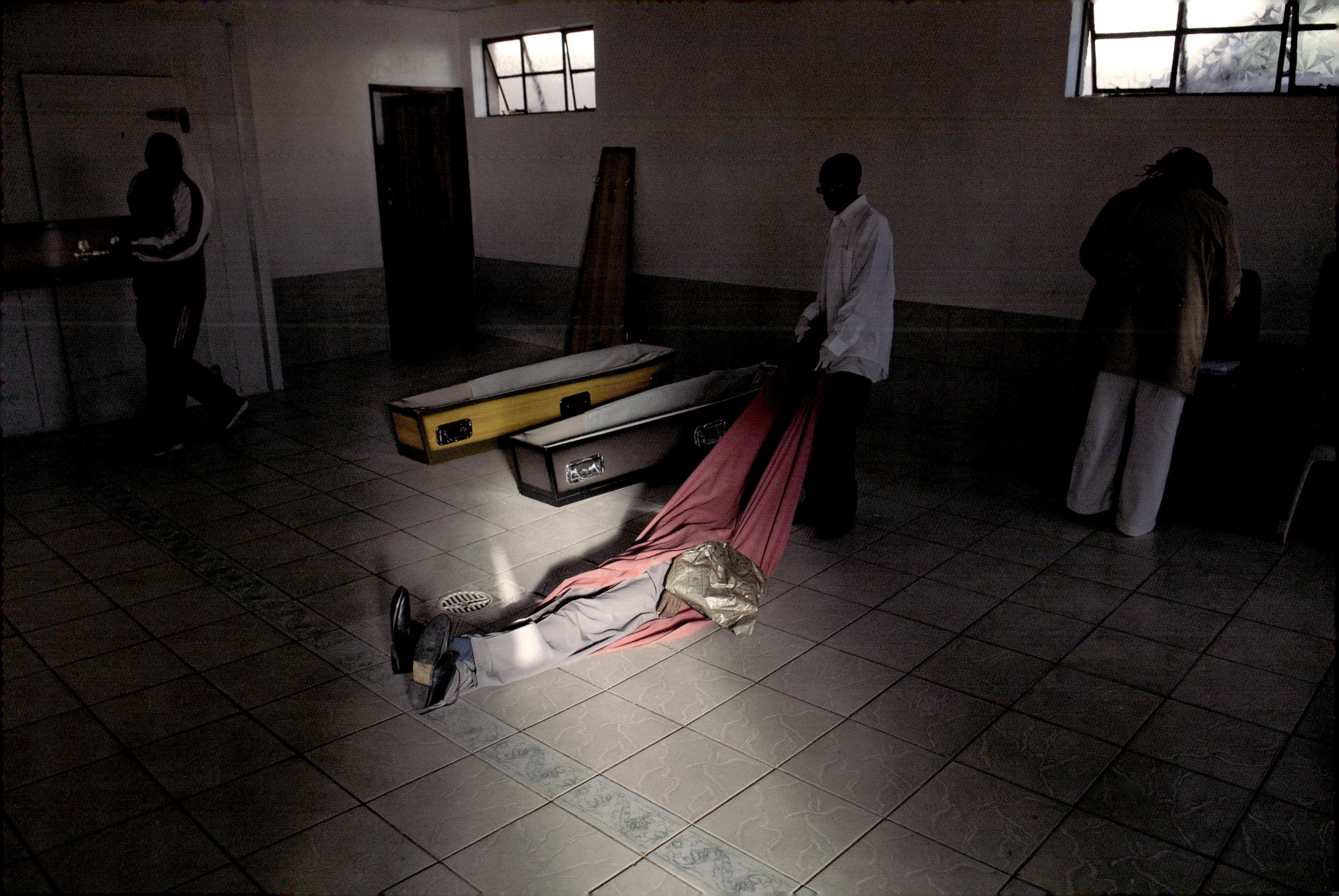

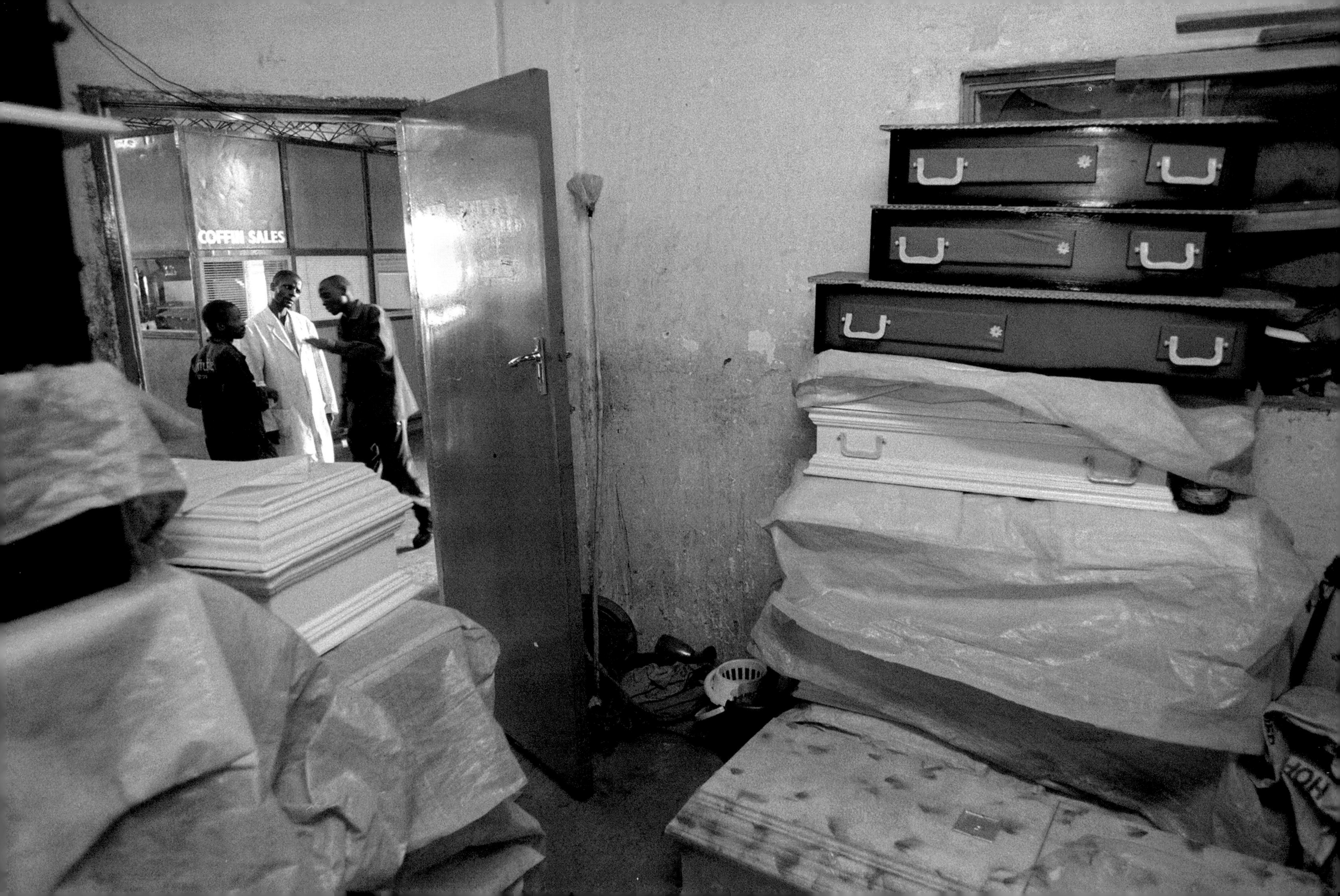

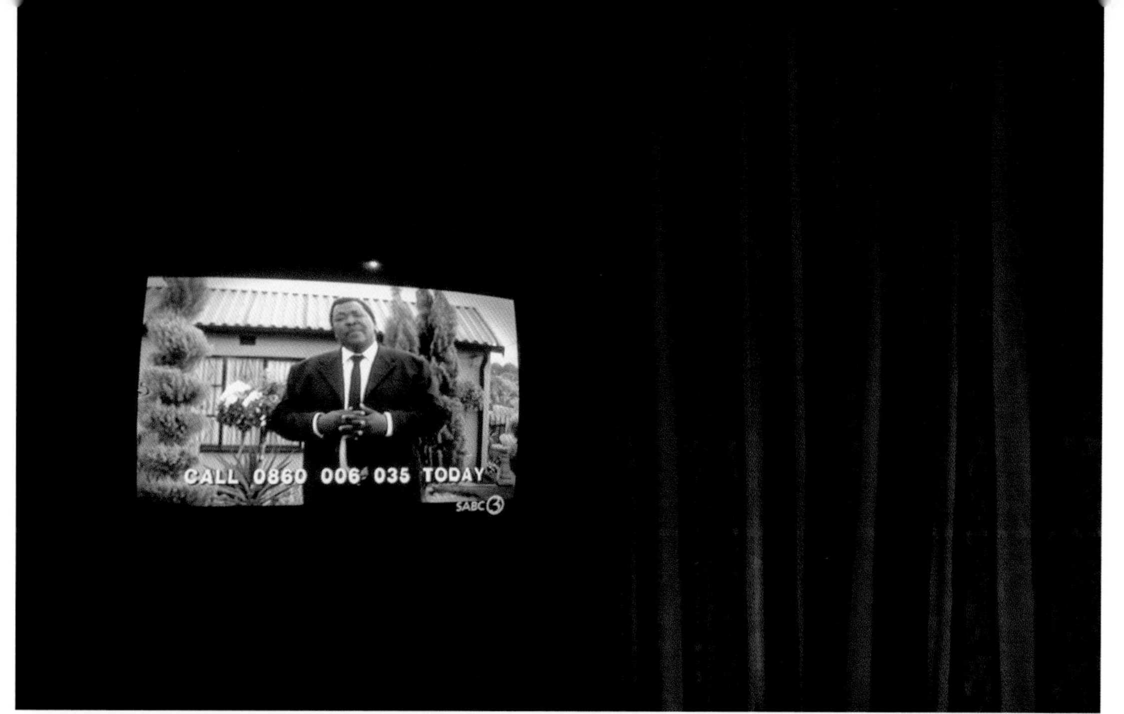
CALL 0860 006 035 TODAY
SABC

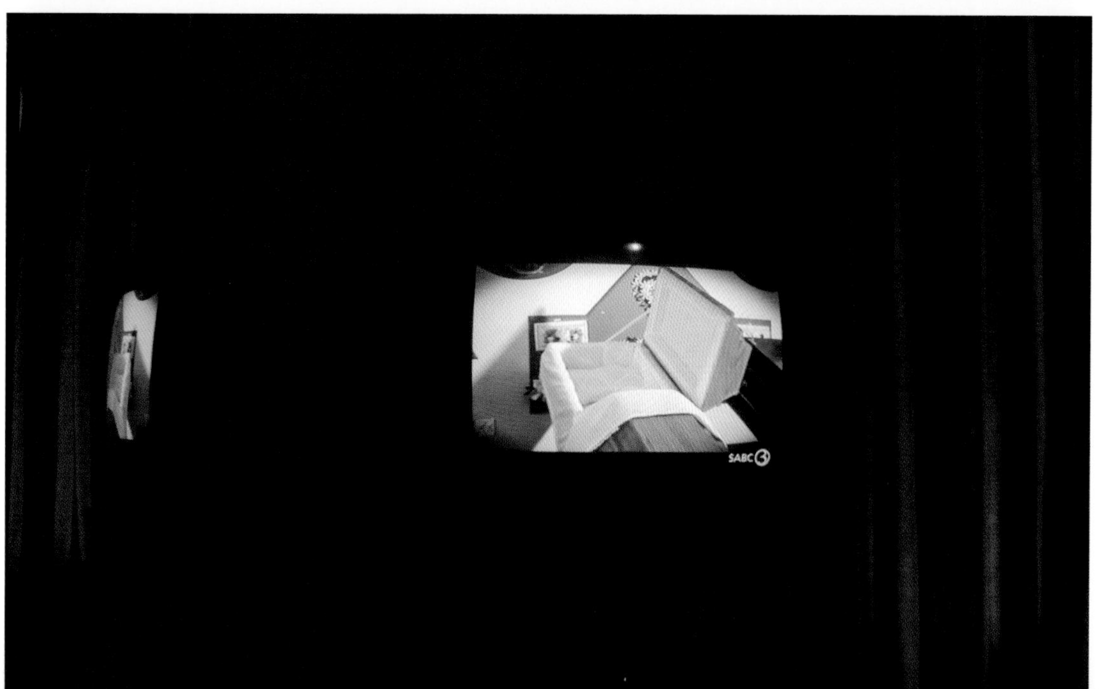
SABC

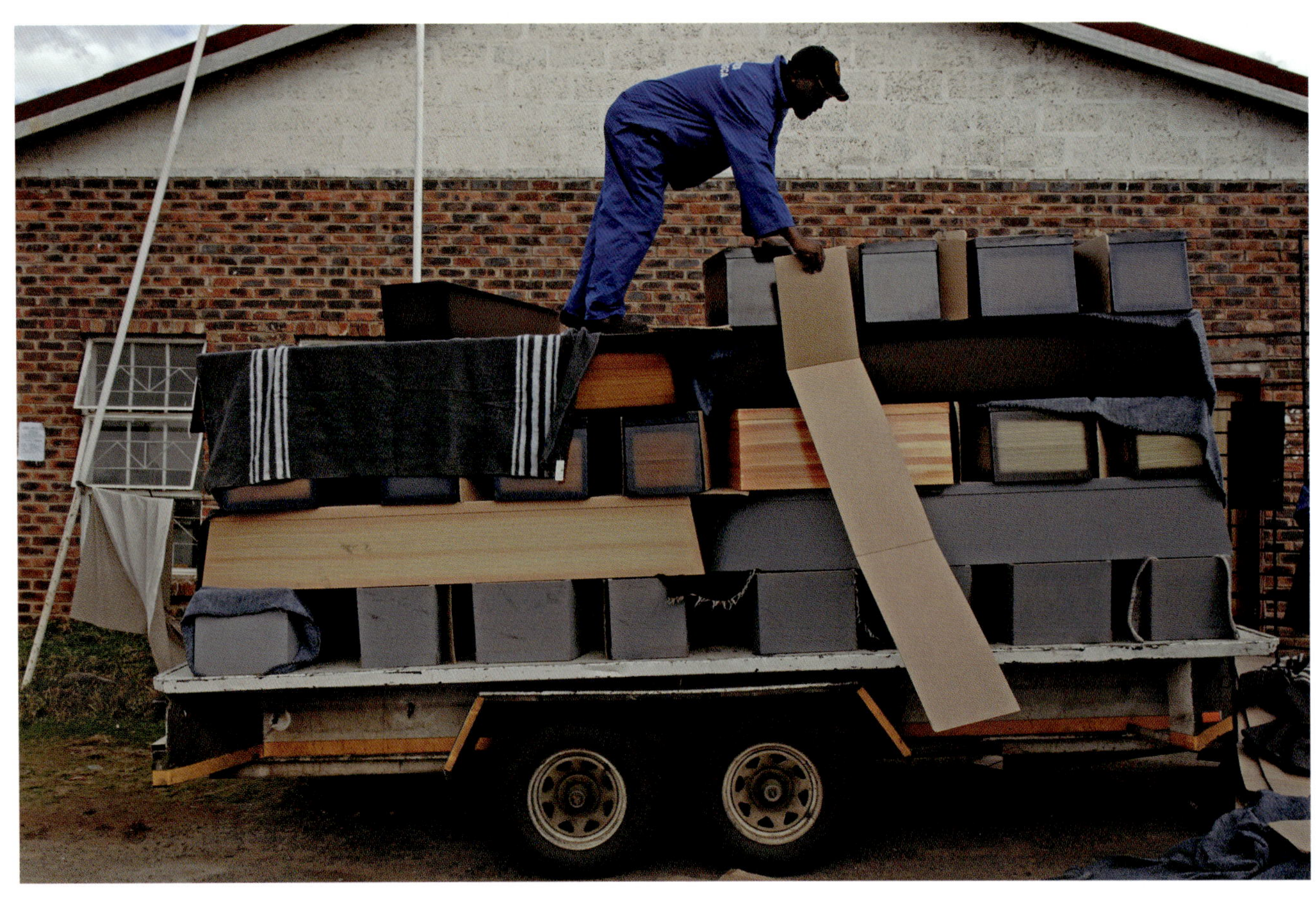

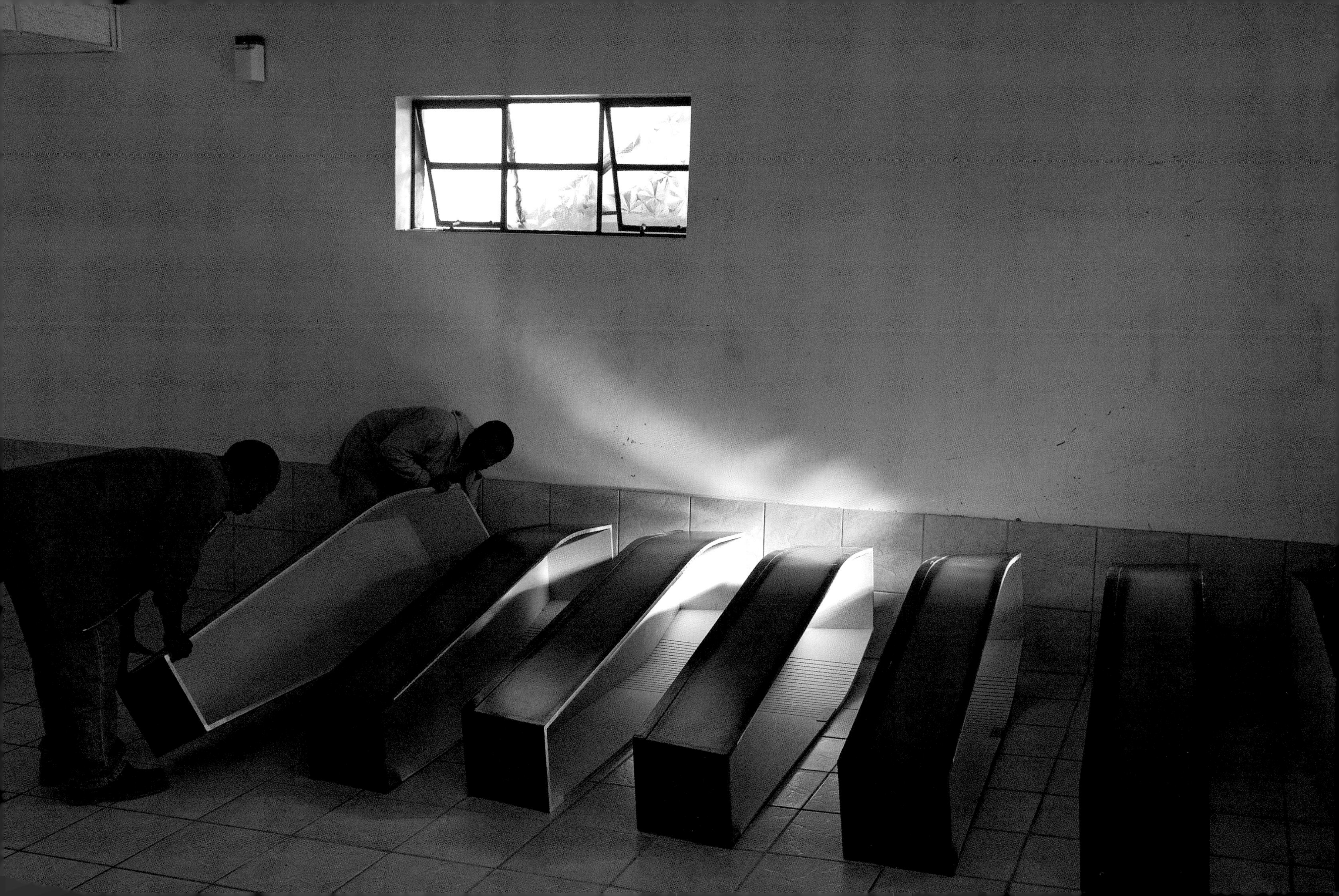

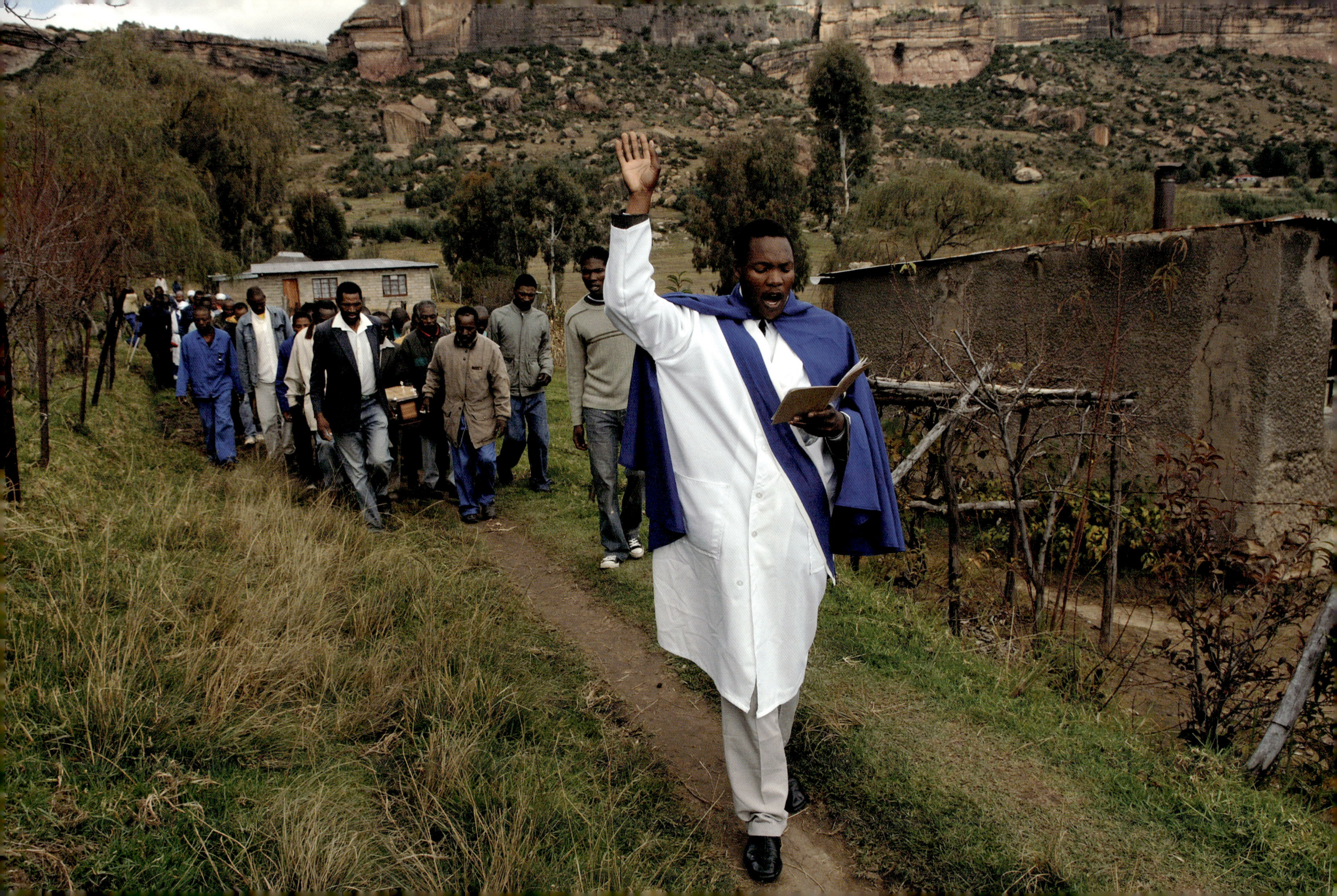

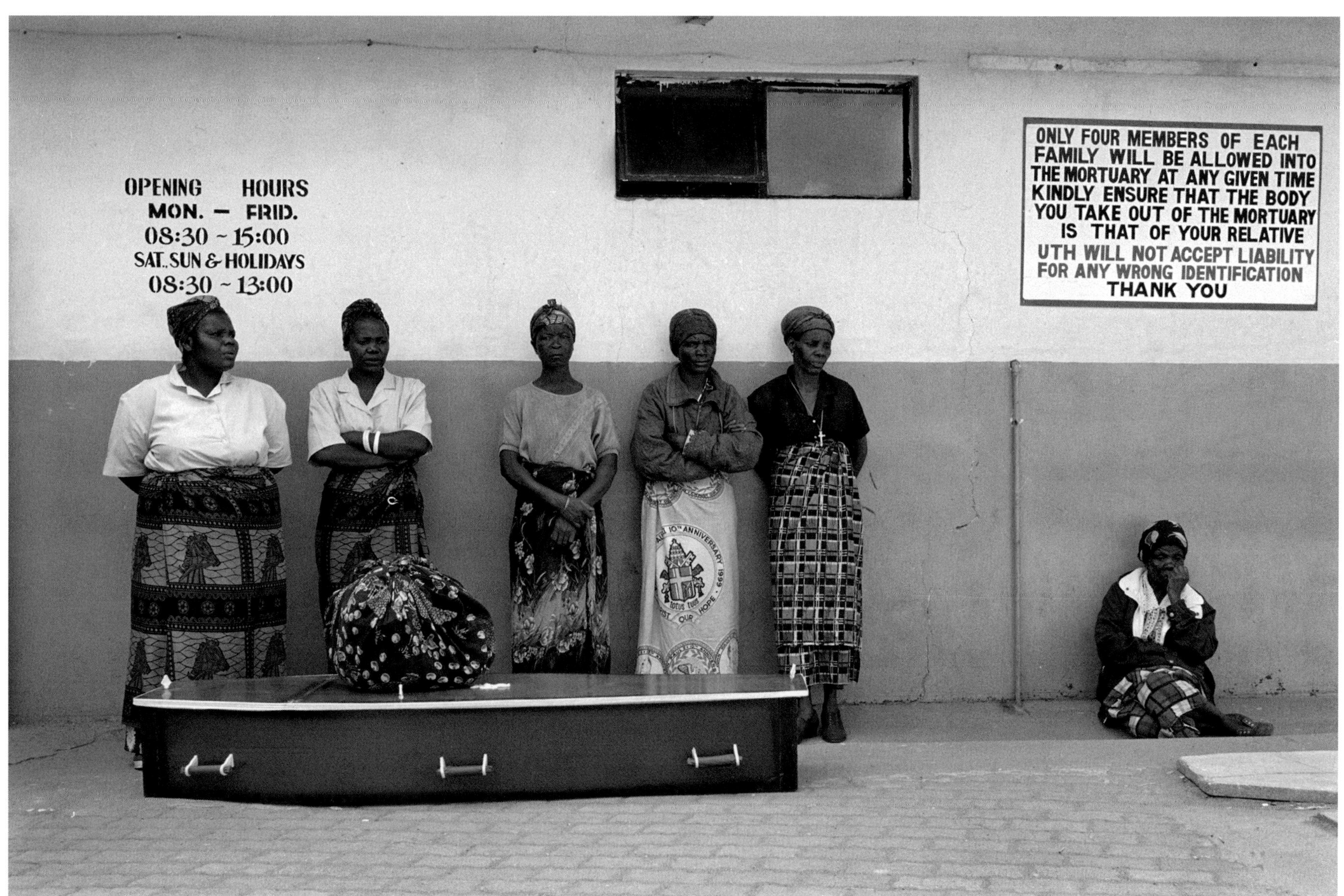

OPENING   HOURS
MON. - FRID.
08:30 ~ 15:00
SAT..SUN & HOLIDAYS
08:30 ~ 13:00
ONLY FOUR MEMBERS OF EACH
FAMILY WILL BE ALLOWED INTO
THE MORTUARY AT ANY GIVEN TIME
KINDLY ENSURE THAT THE BODY
YOU TAKE OUT OF THE MORTUARY
IS THAT OF YOUR RELATIVE
UTH WILL NOT ACCEPT LIABILITY
FOR ANY WRONG IDENTIFICATION
THANK YOU

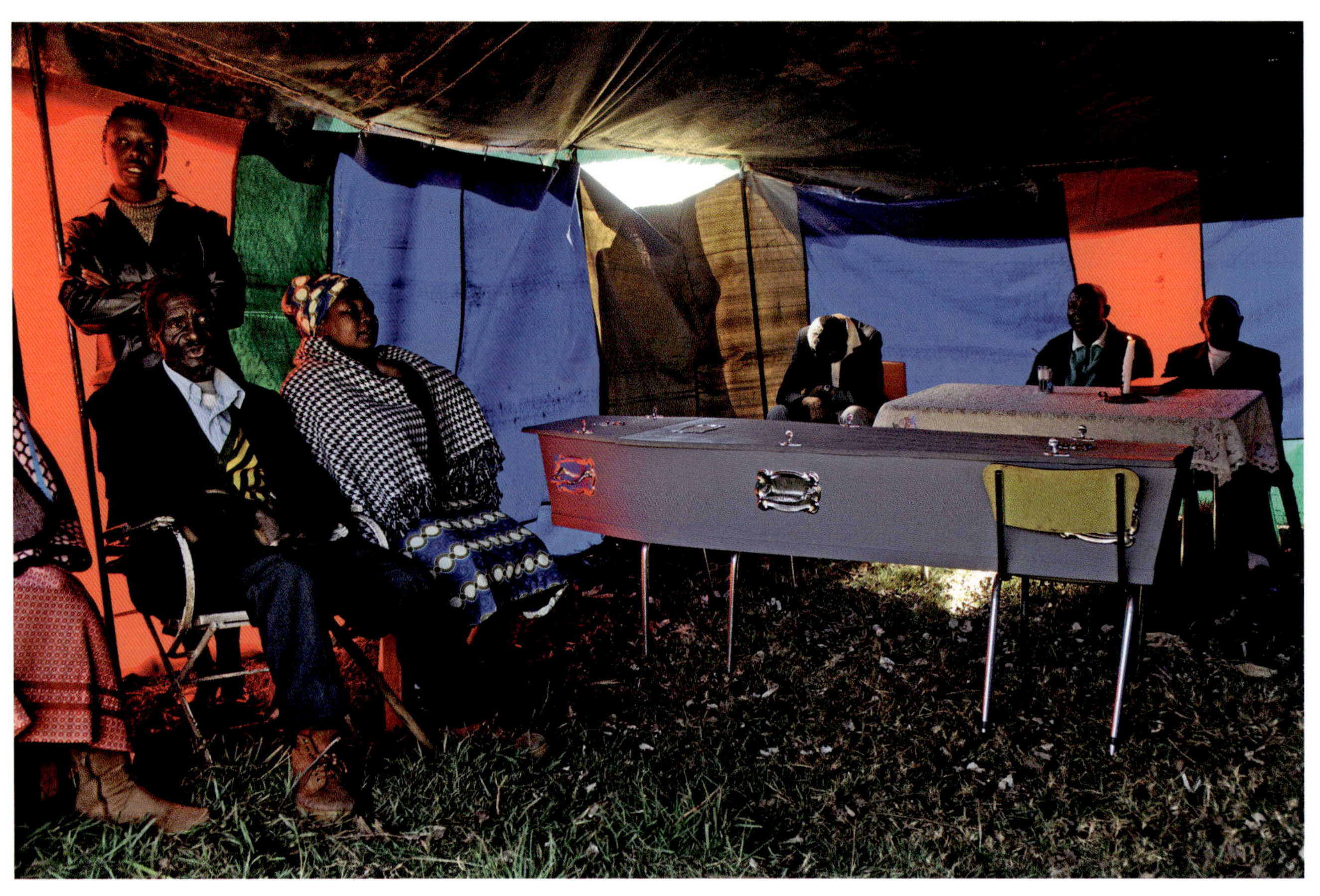

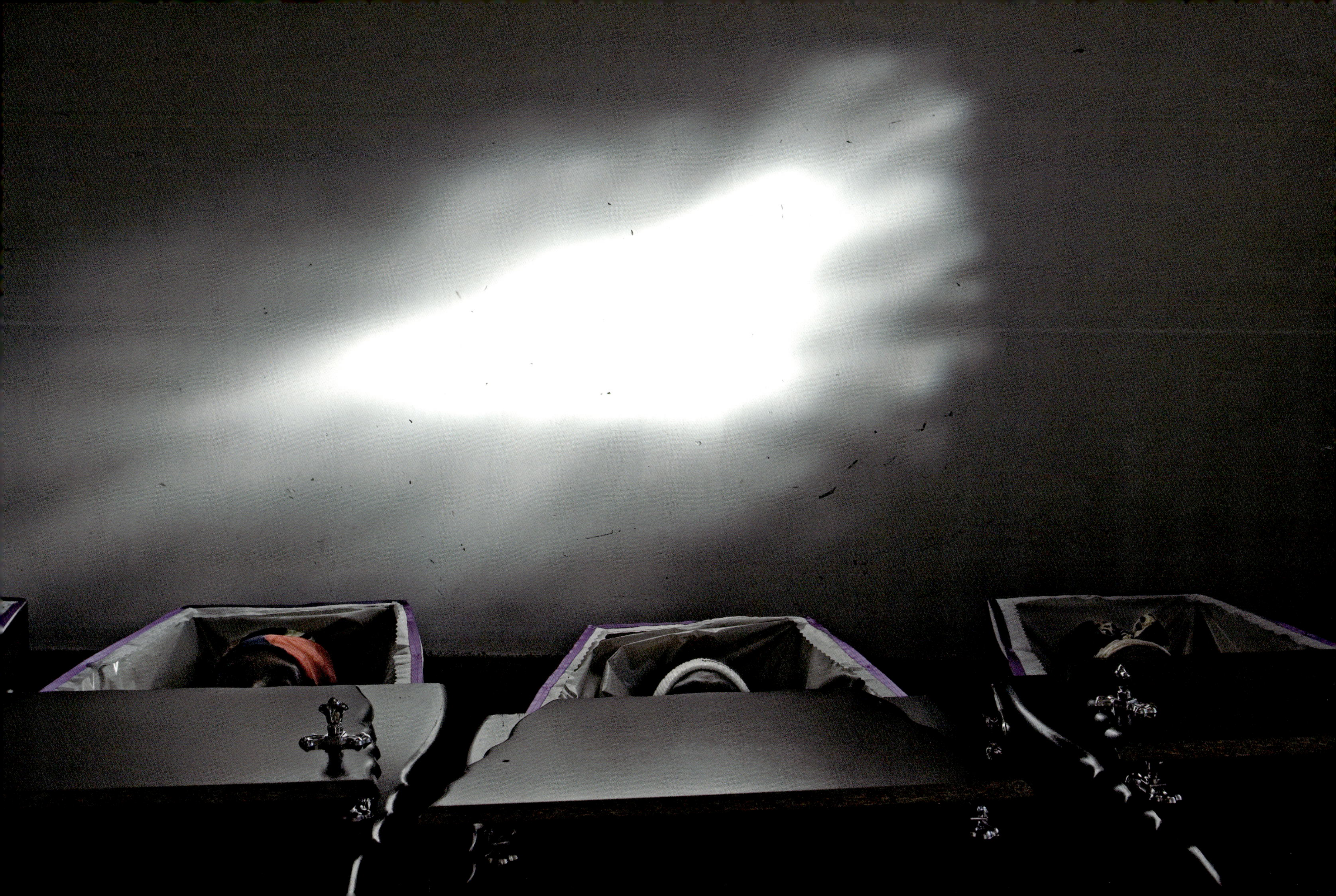

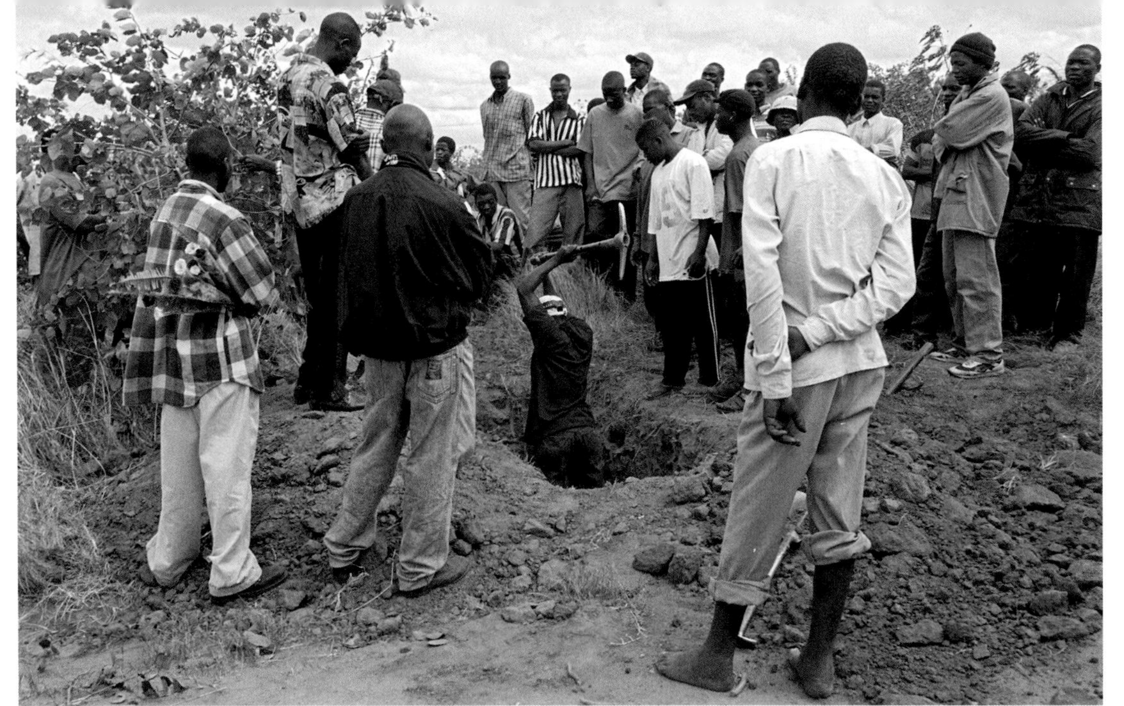

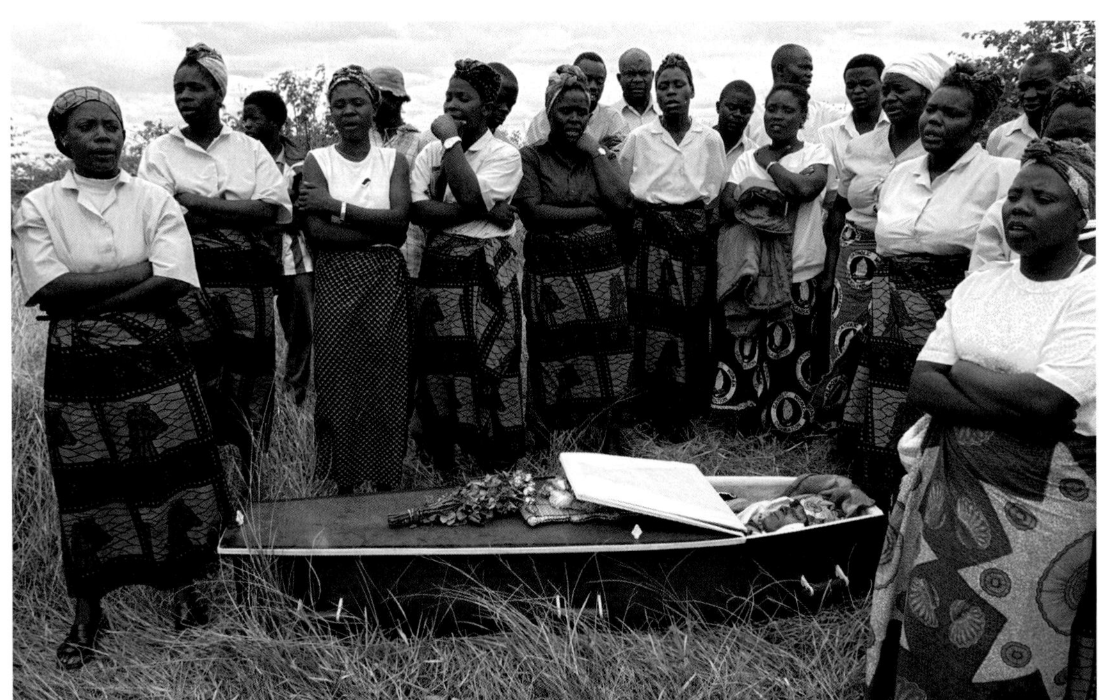

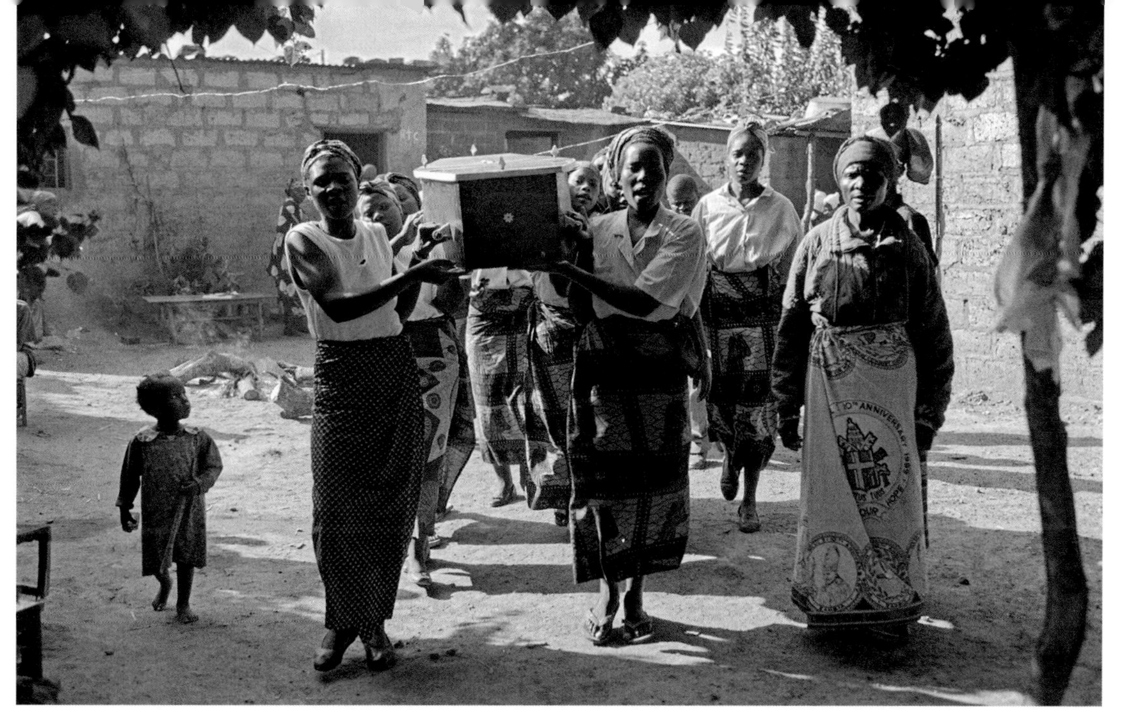

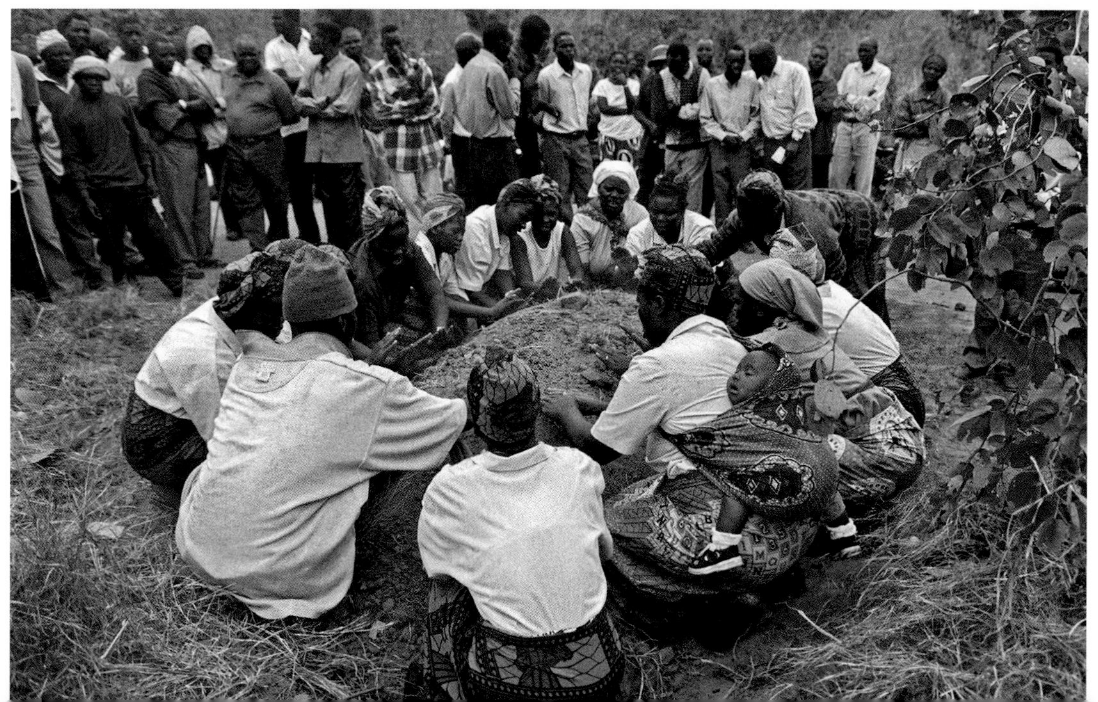

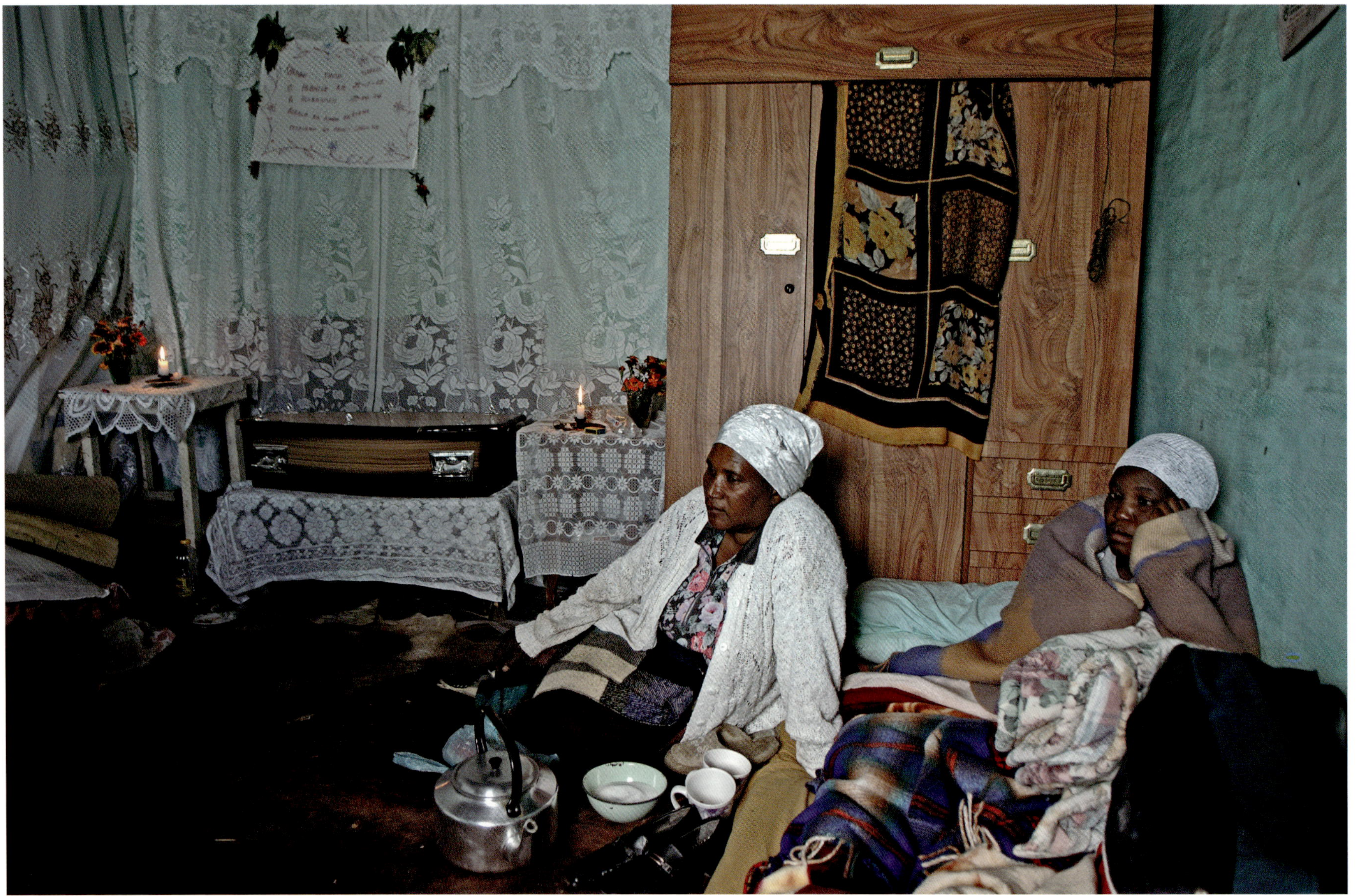

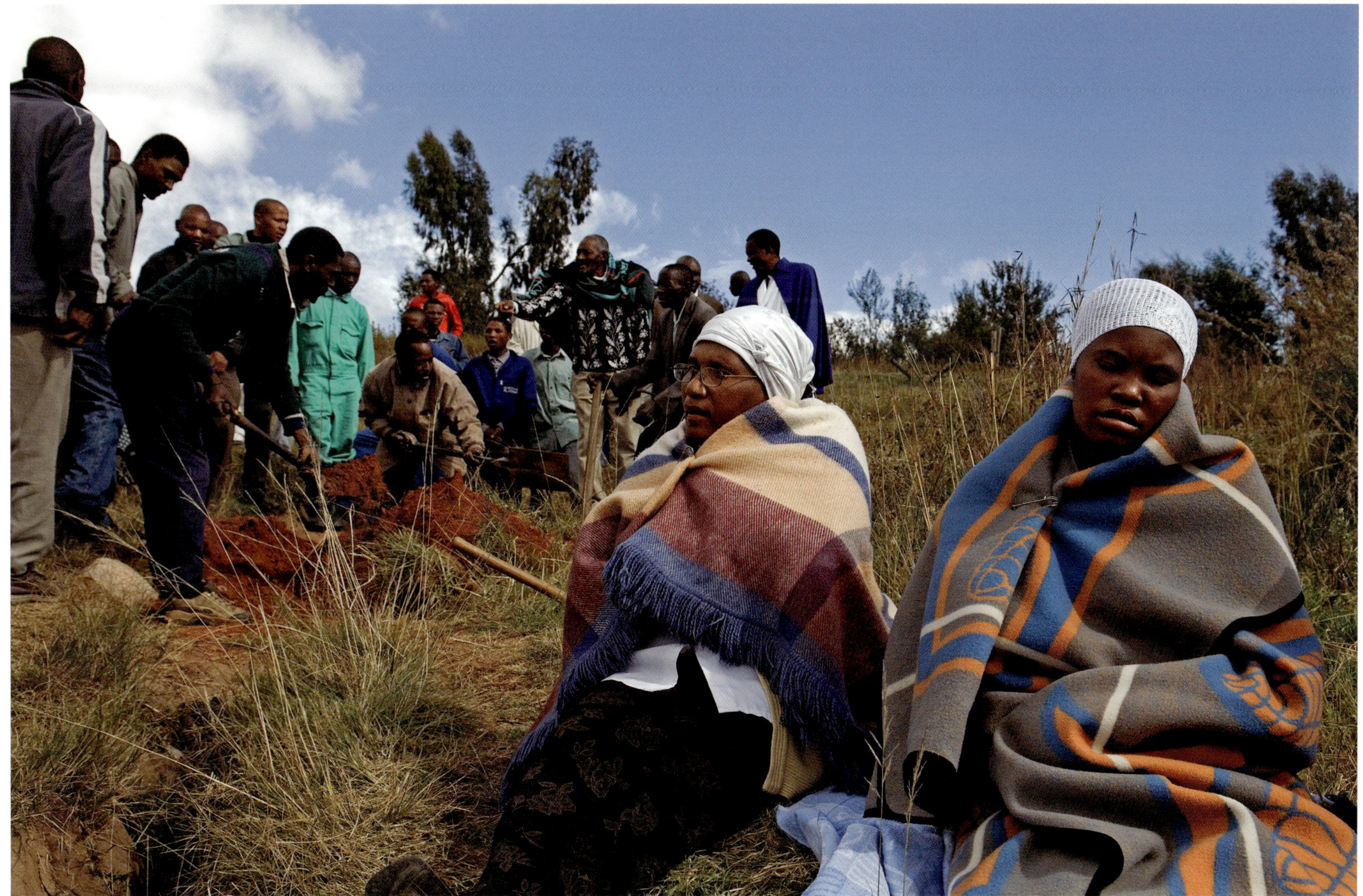

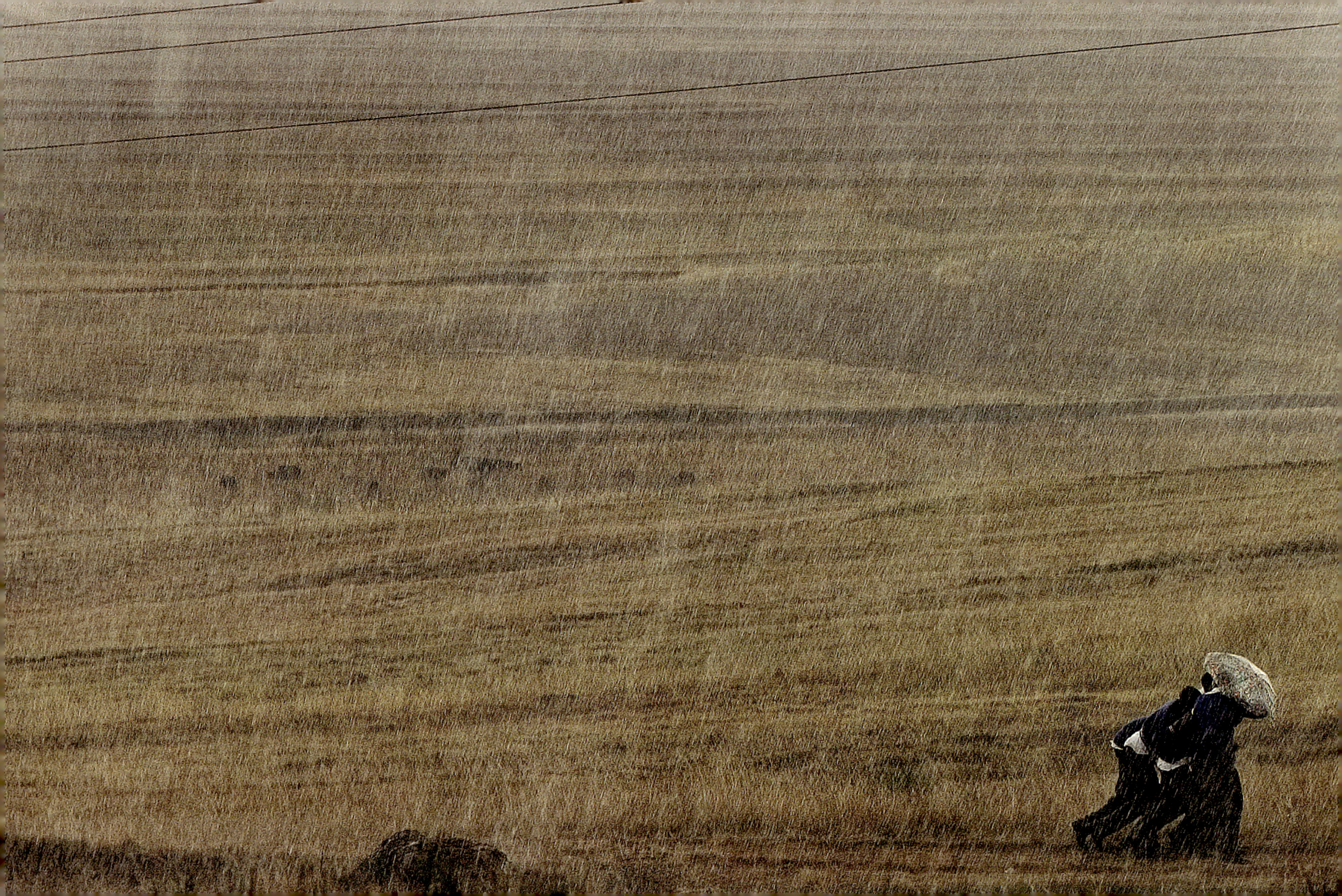

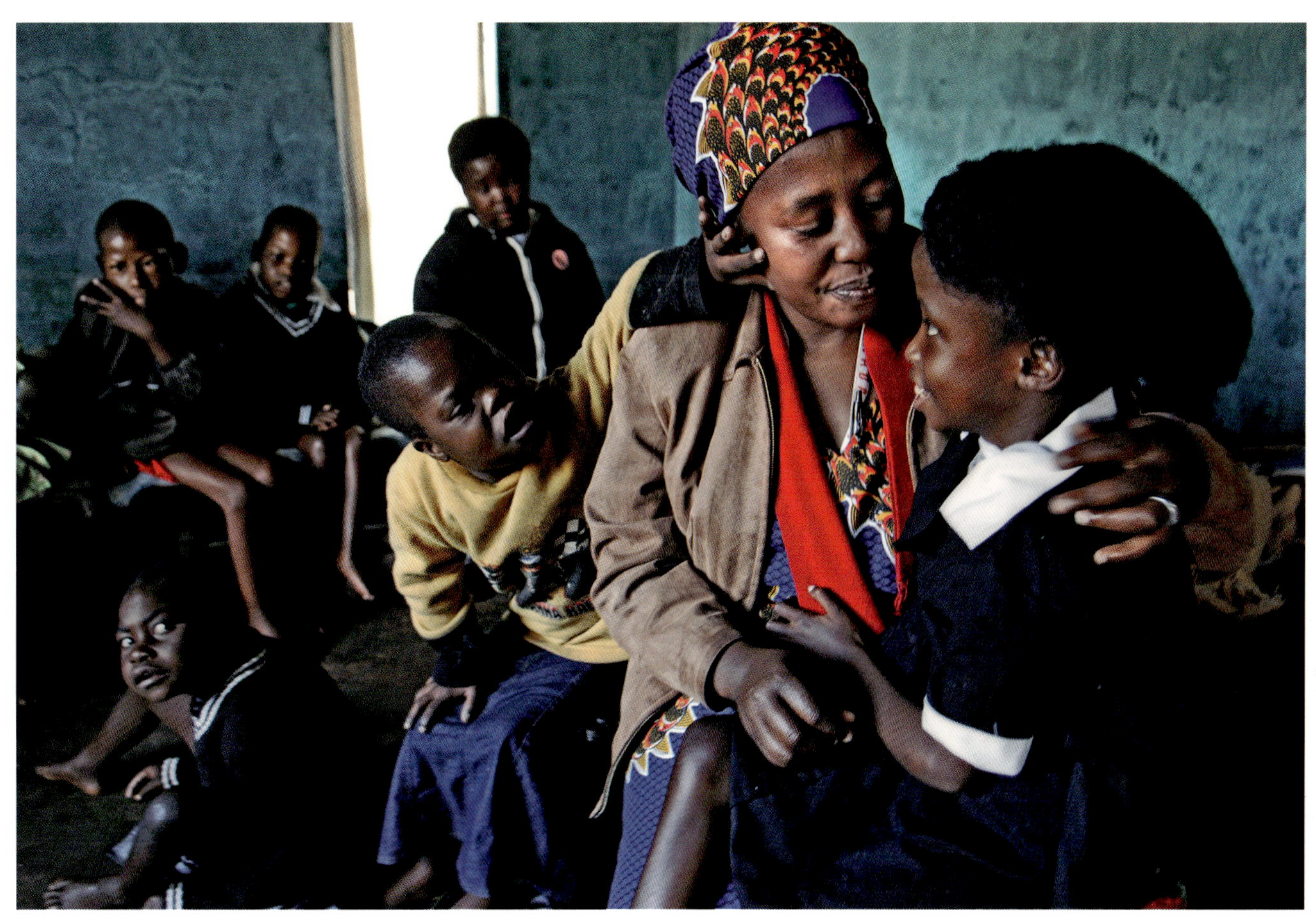

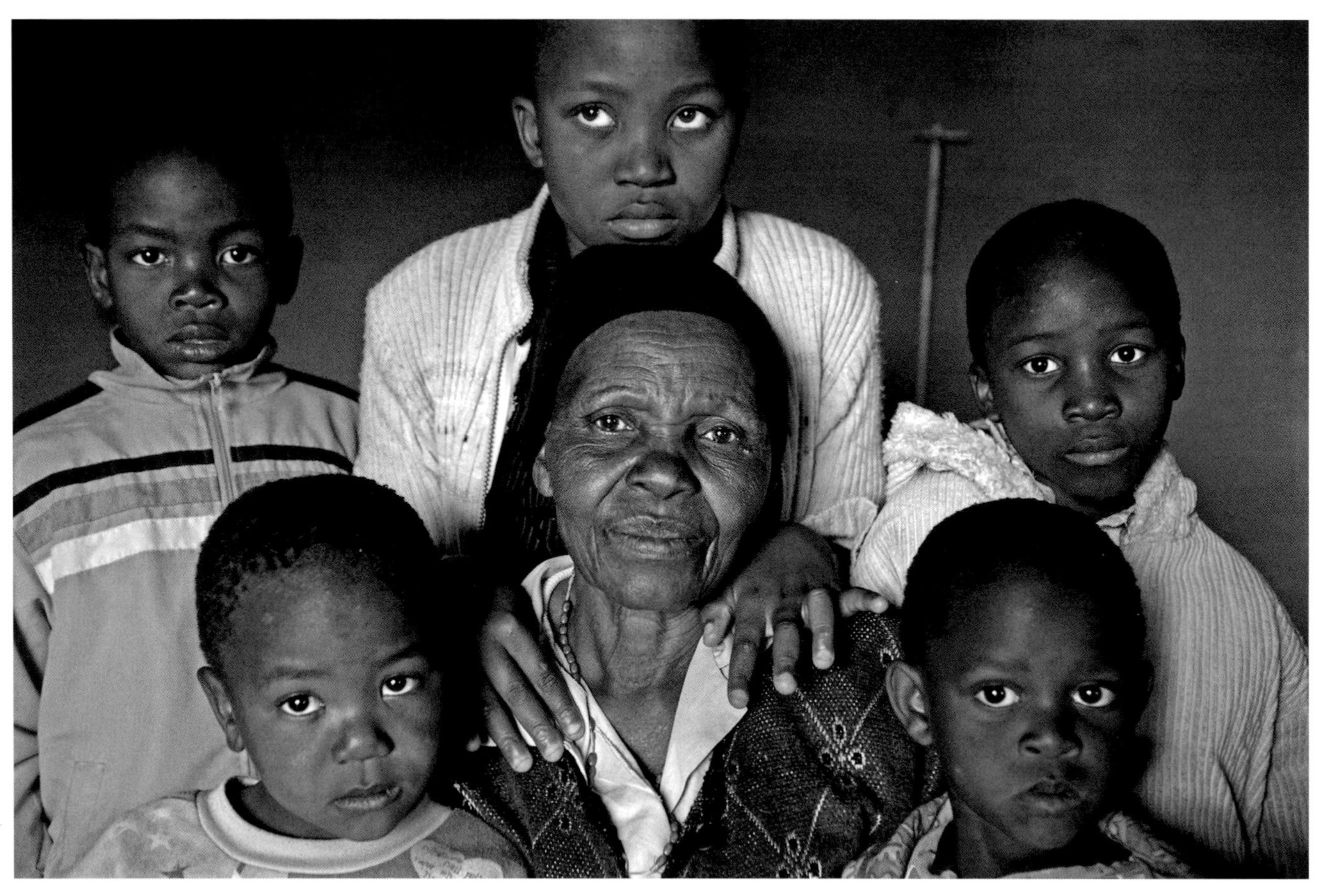

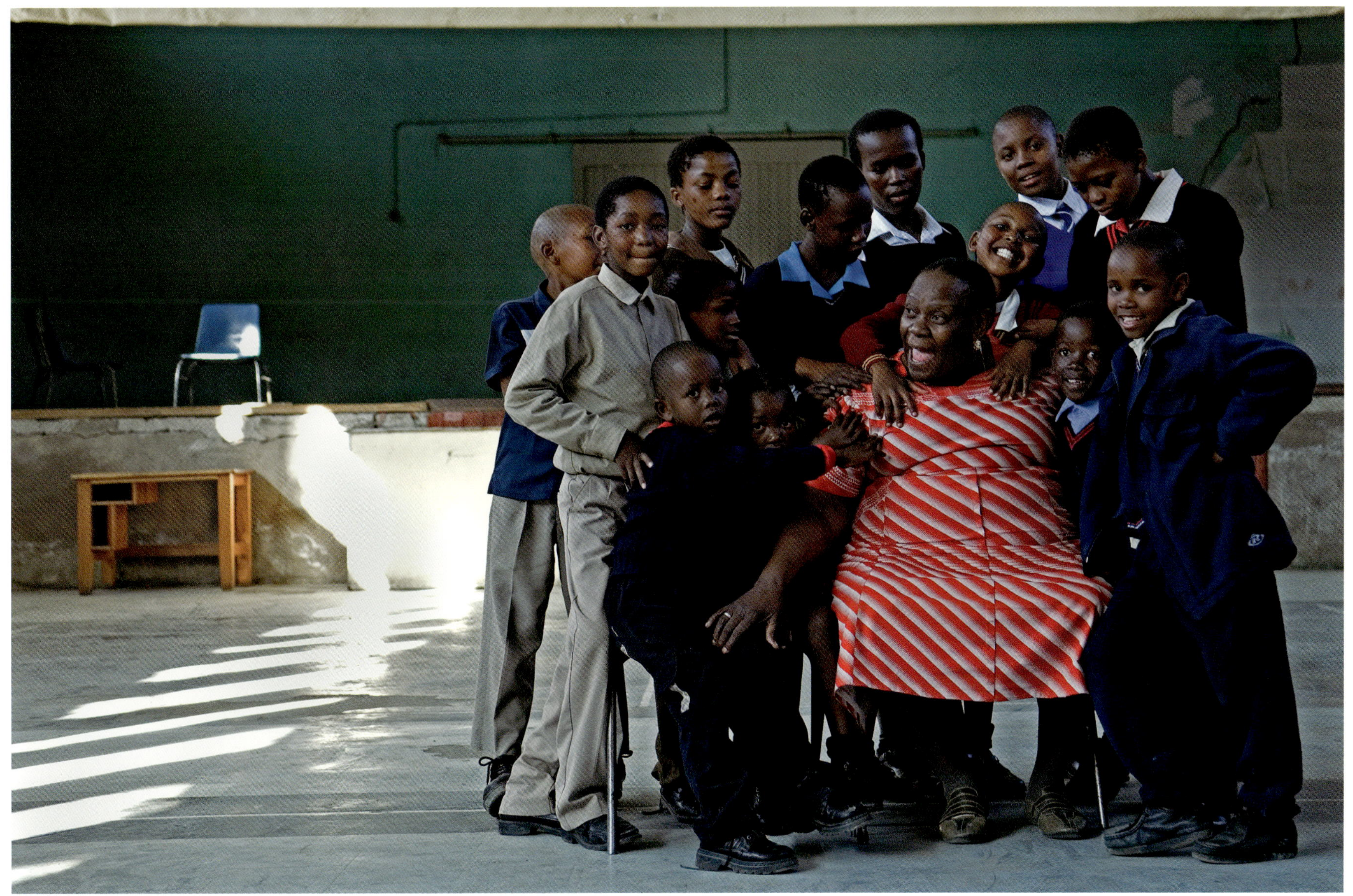

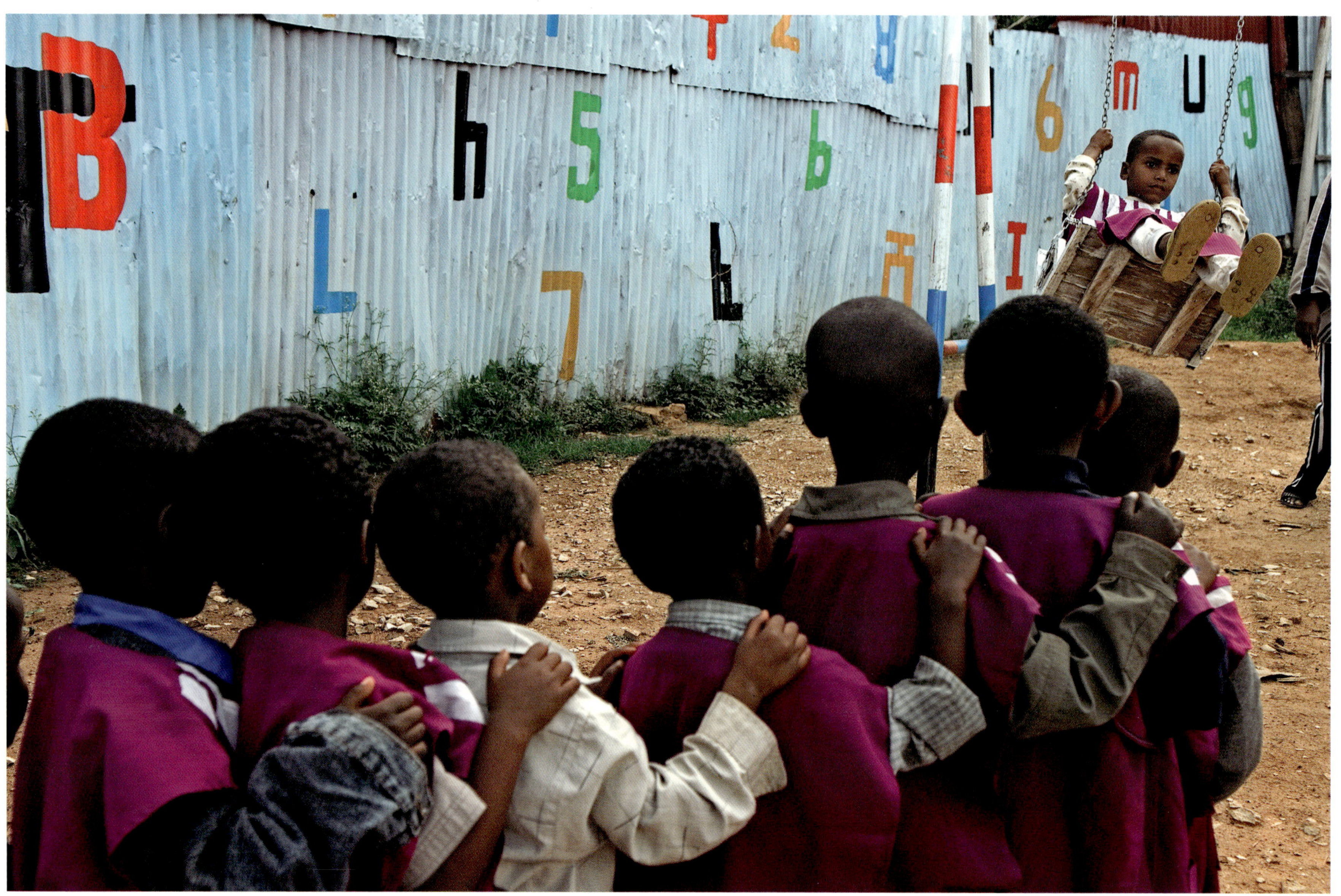

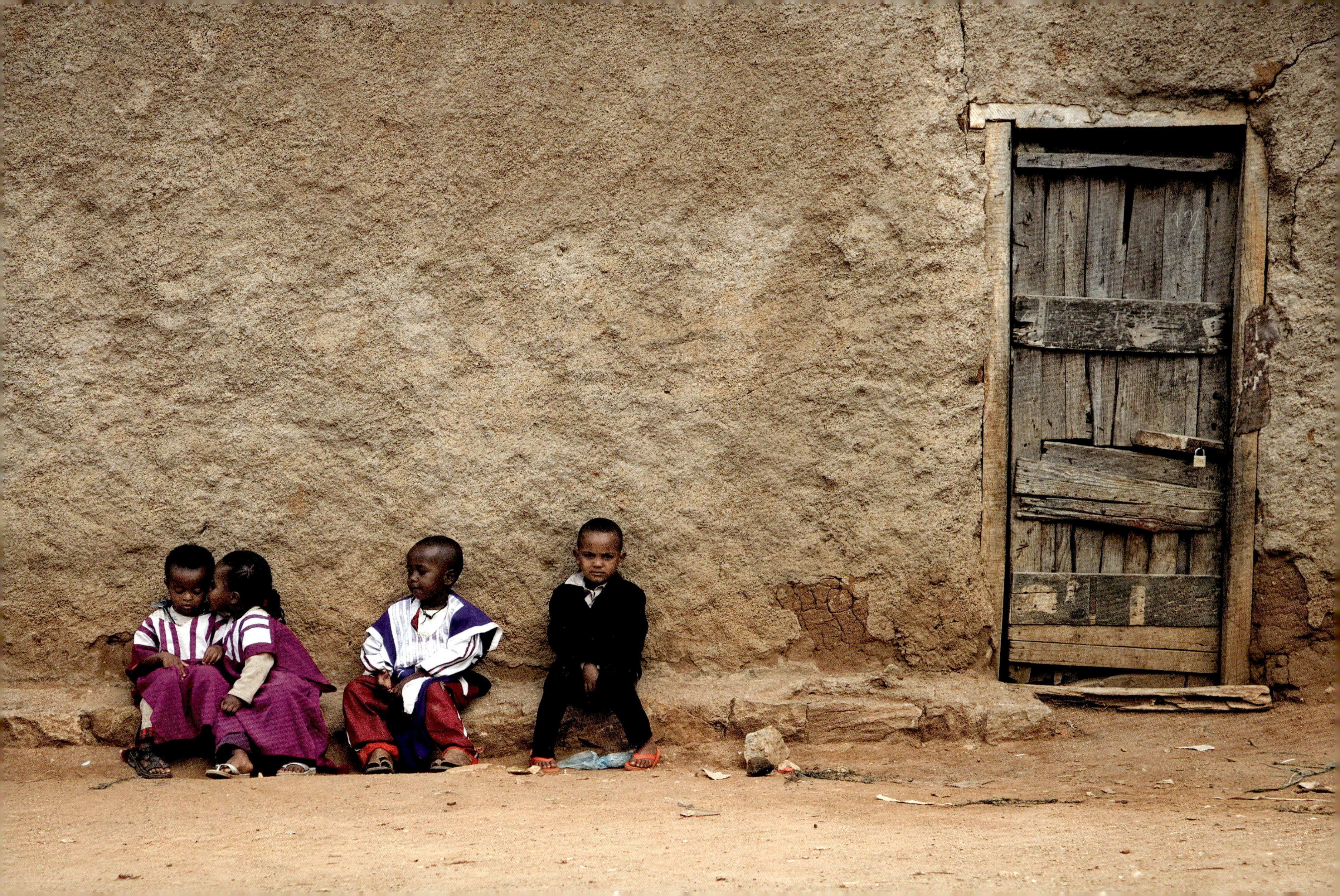

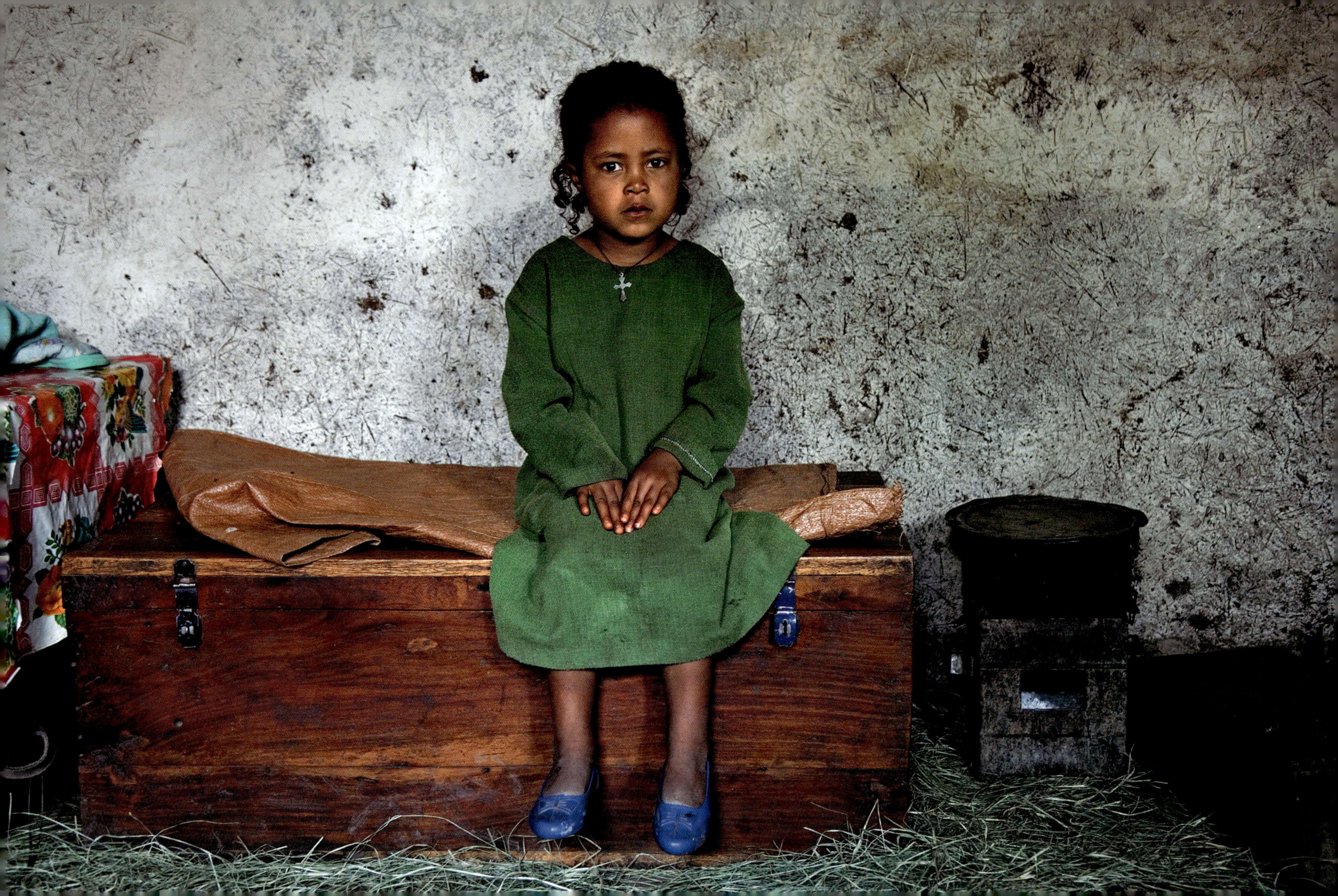

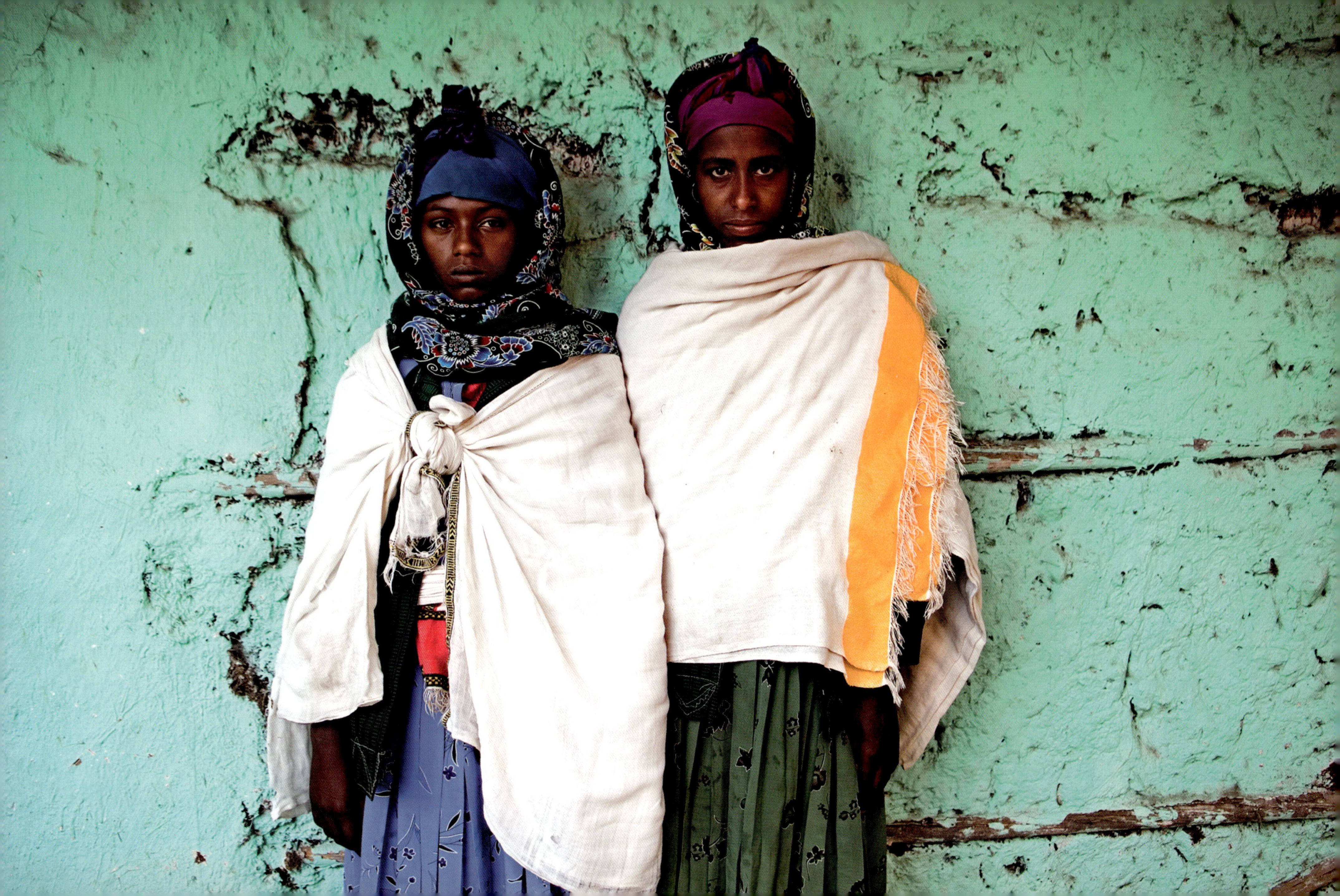

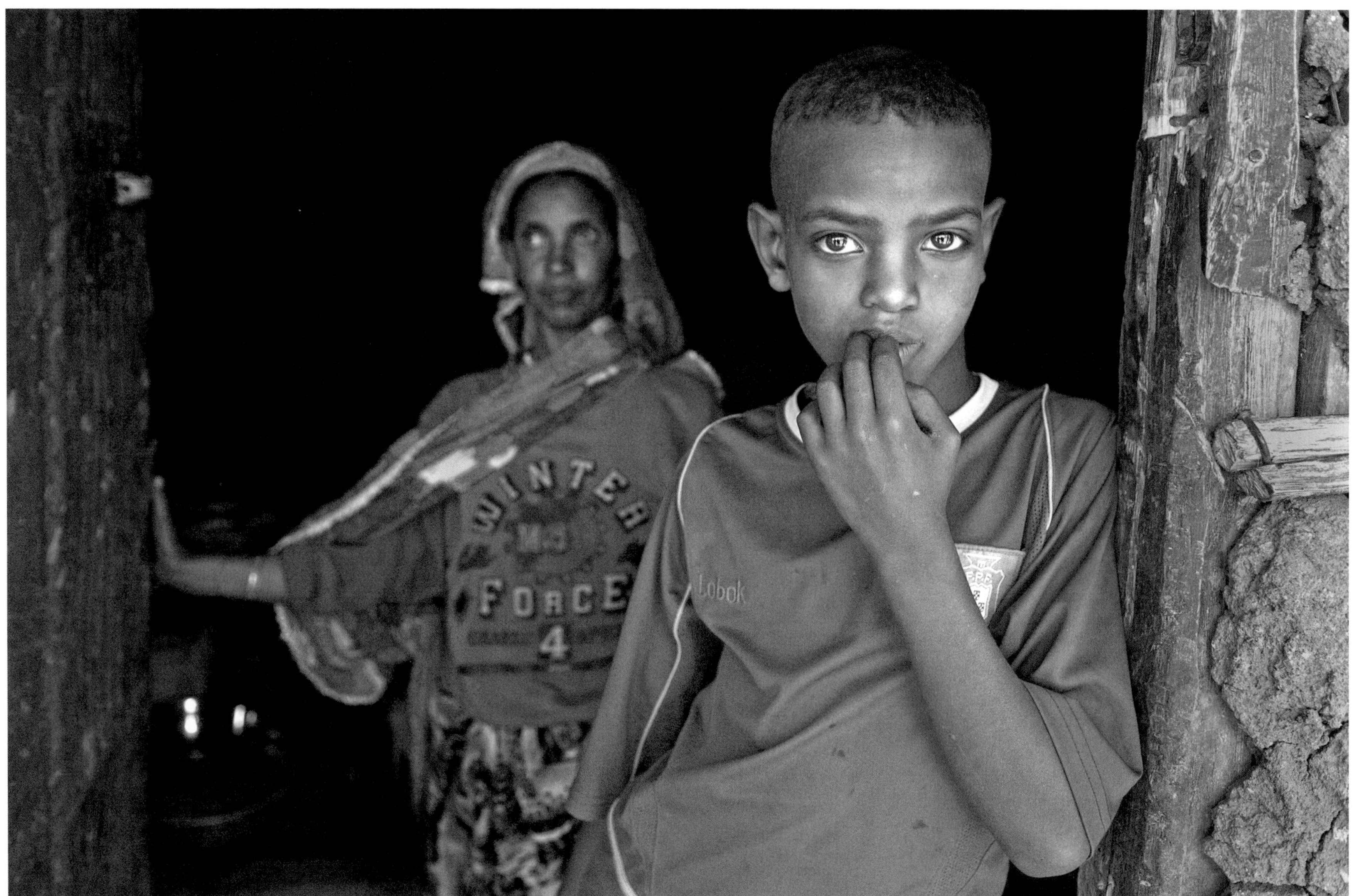

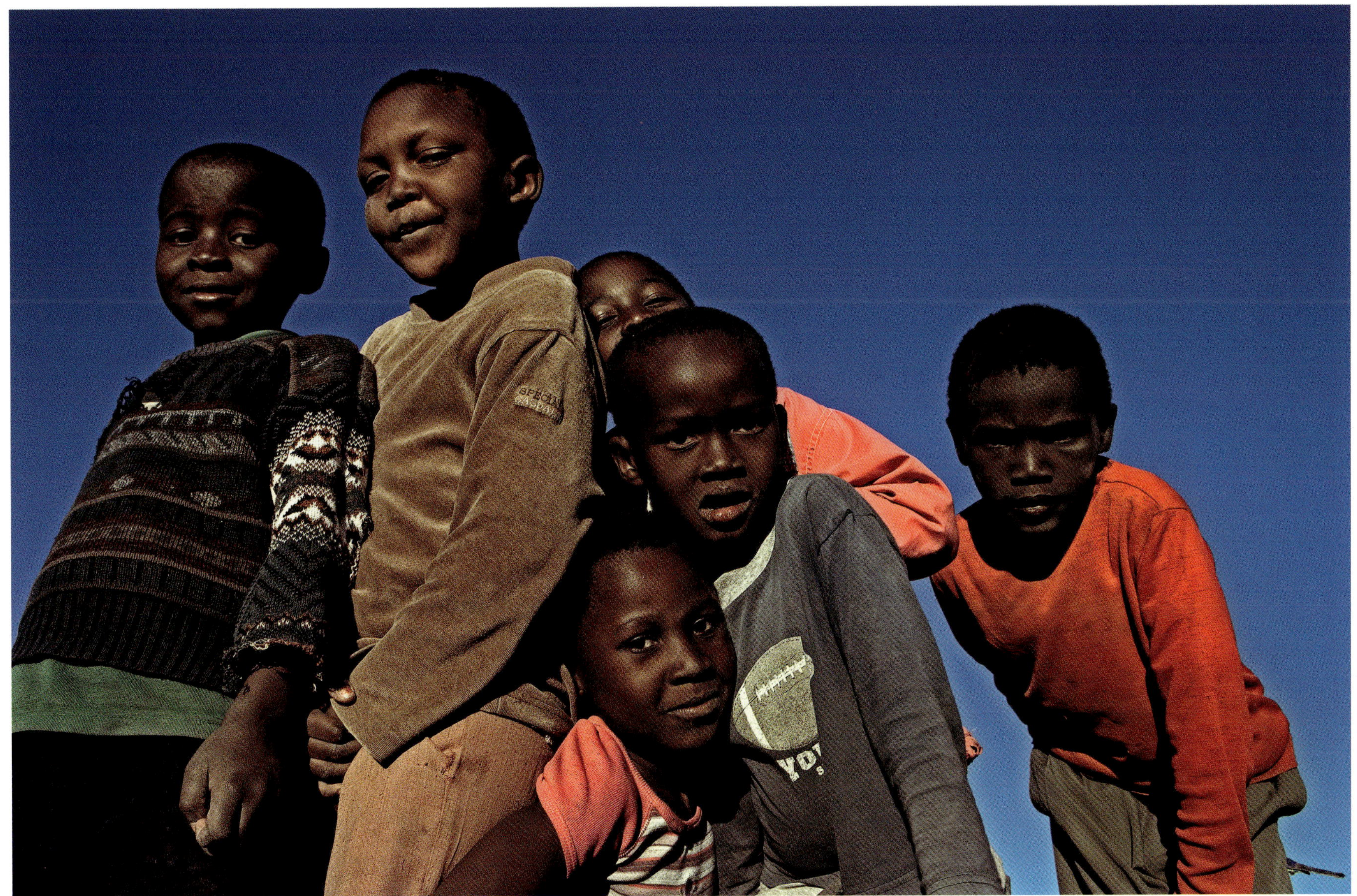

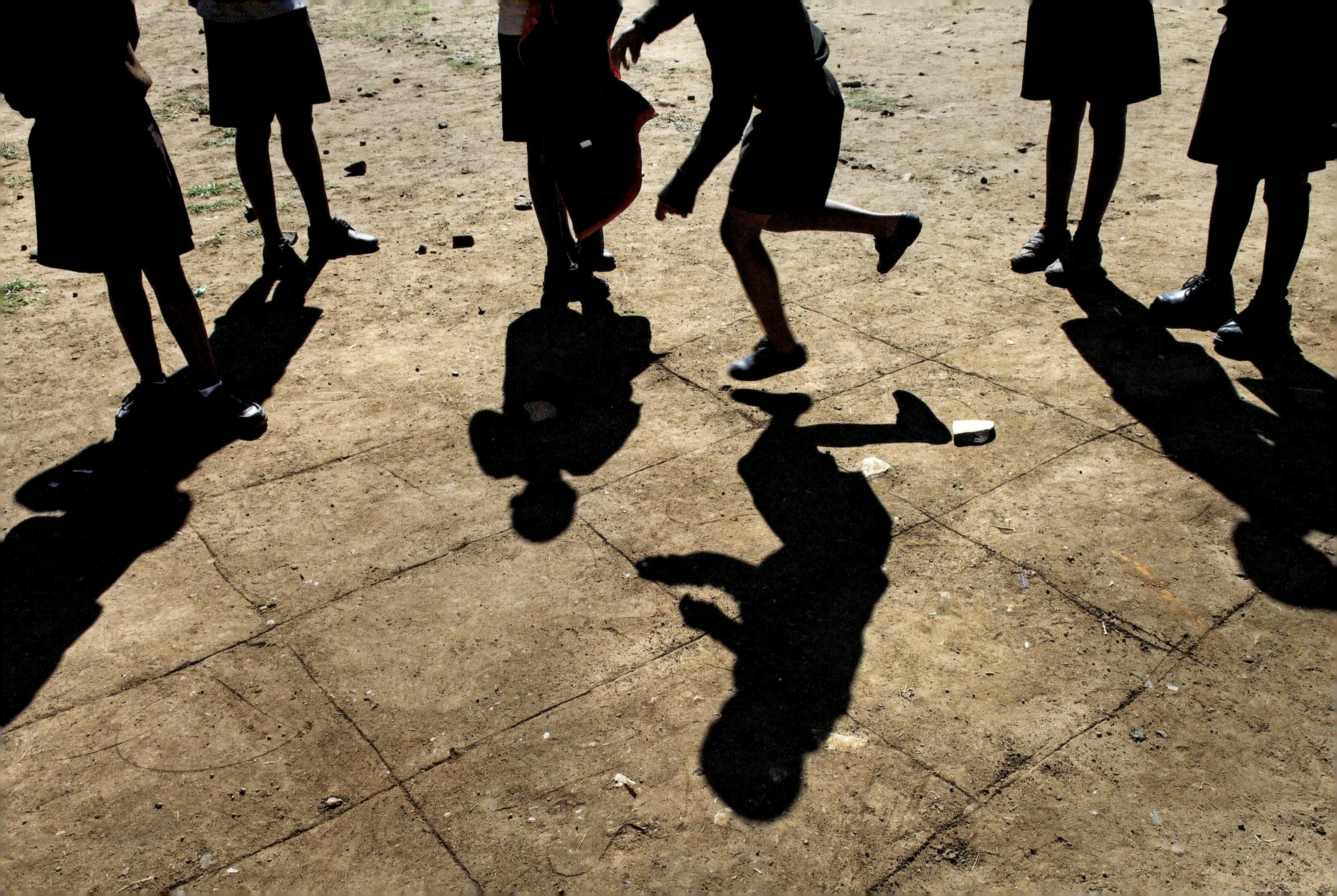

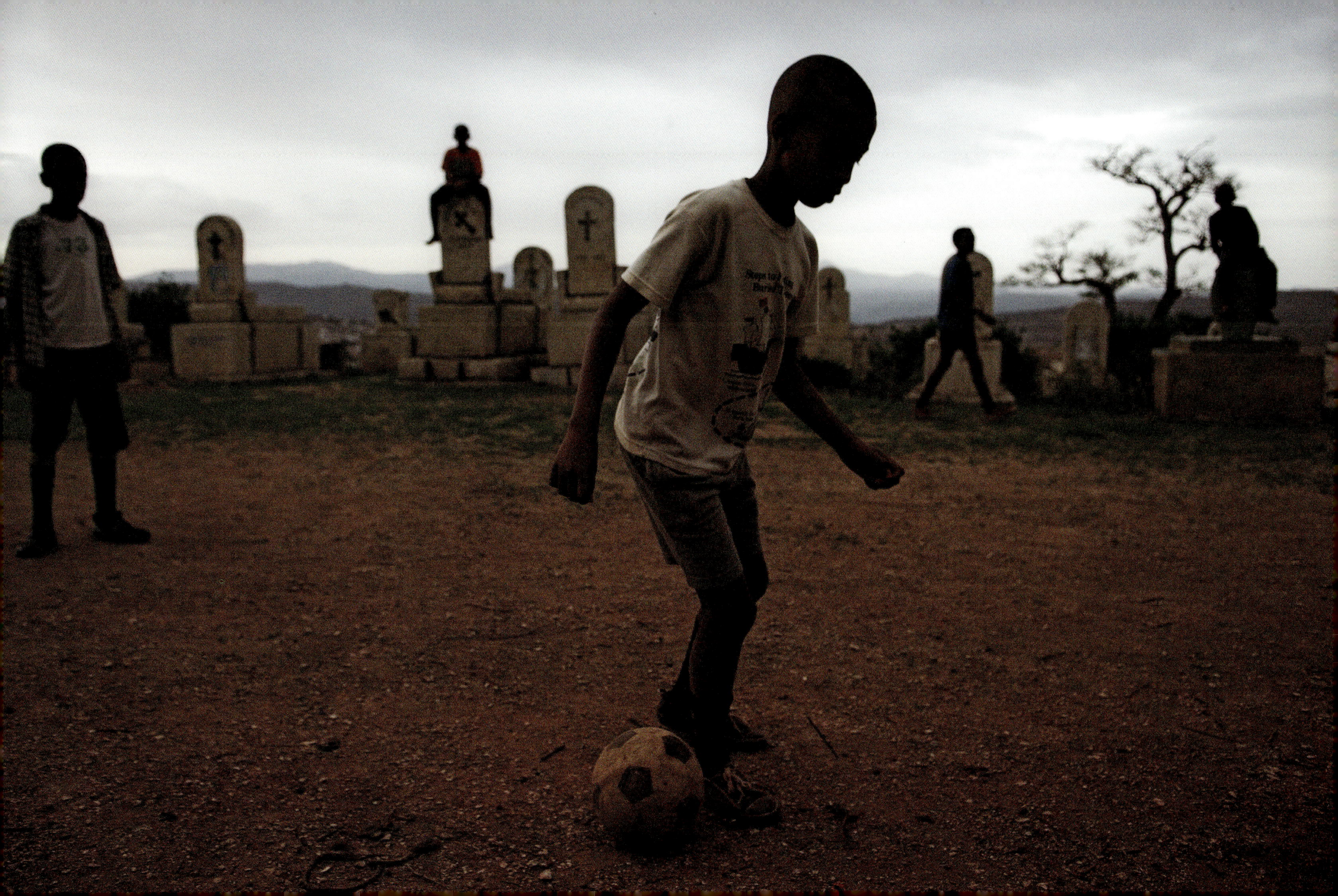

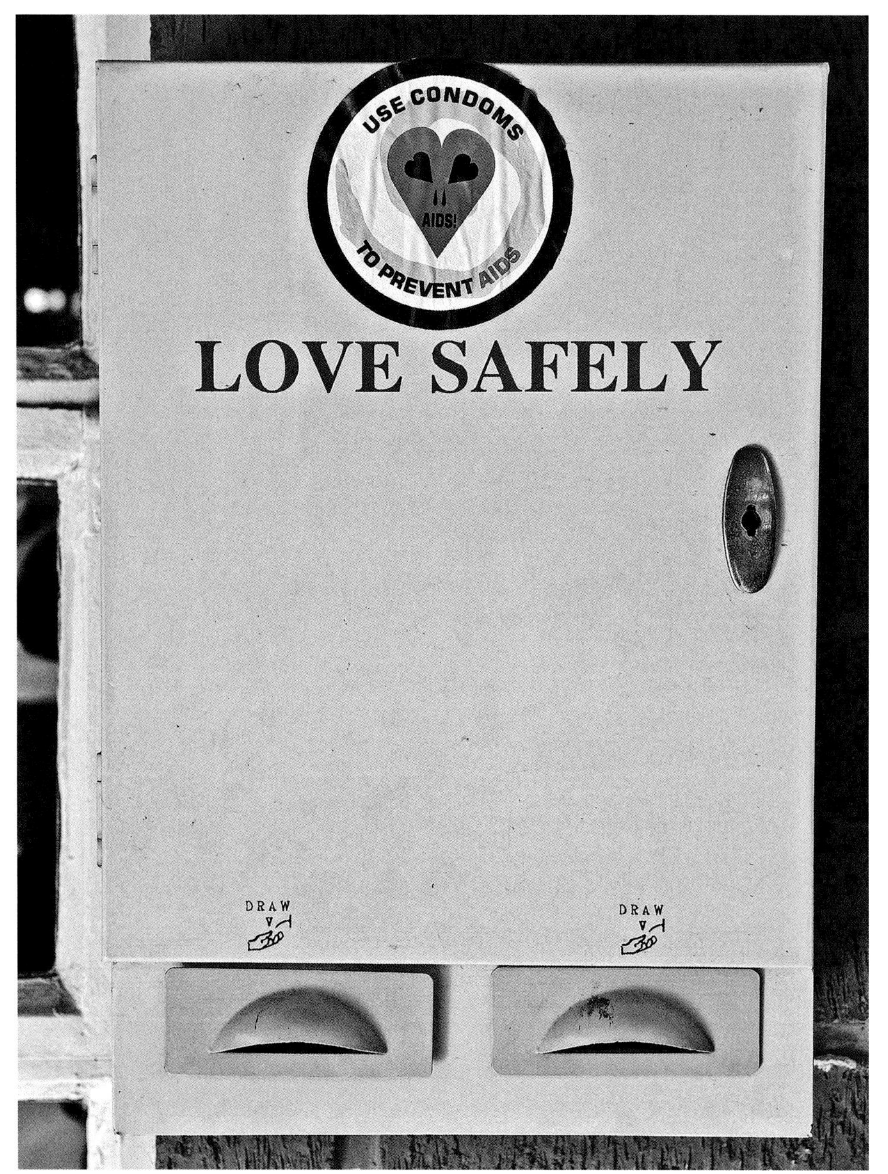

USE CONDOMS
TO PREVENT AIDS
AIDS!
LOVE SAFELY
DRAW
DRAW

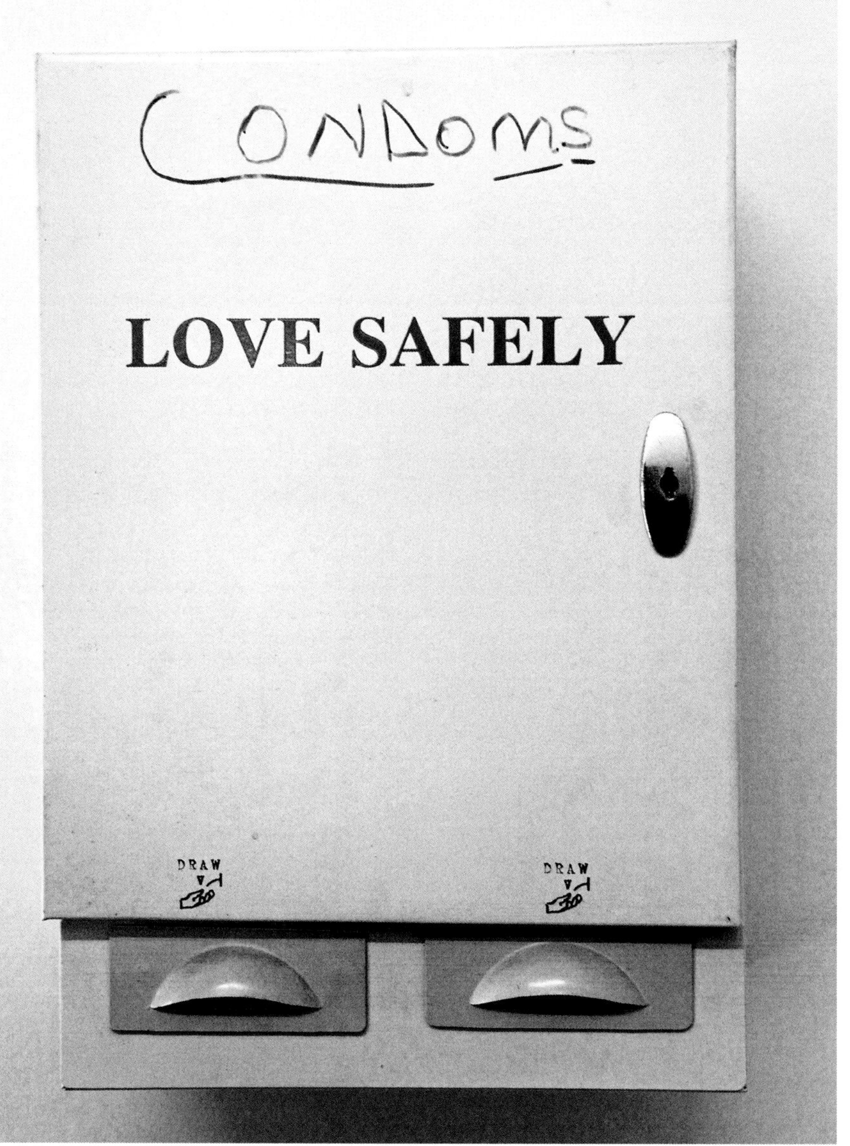

CONDOMS
LOVE SAFELY
DRAW
DRAW

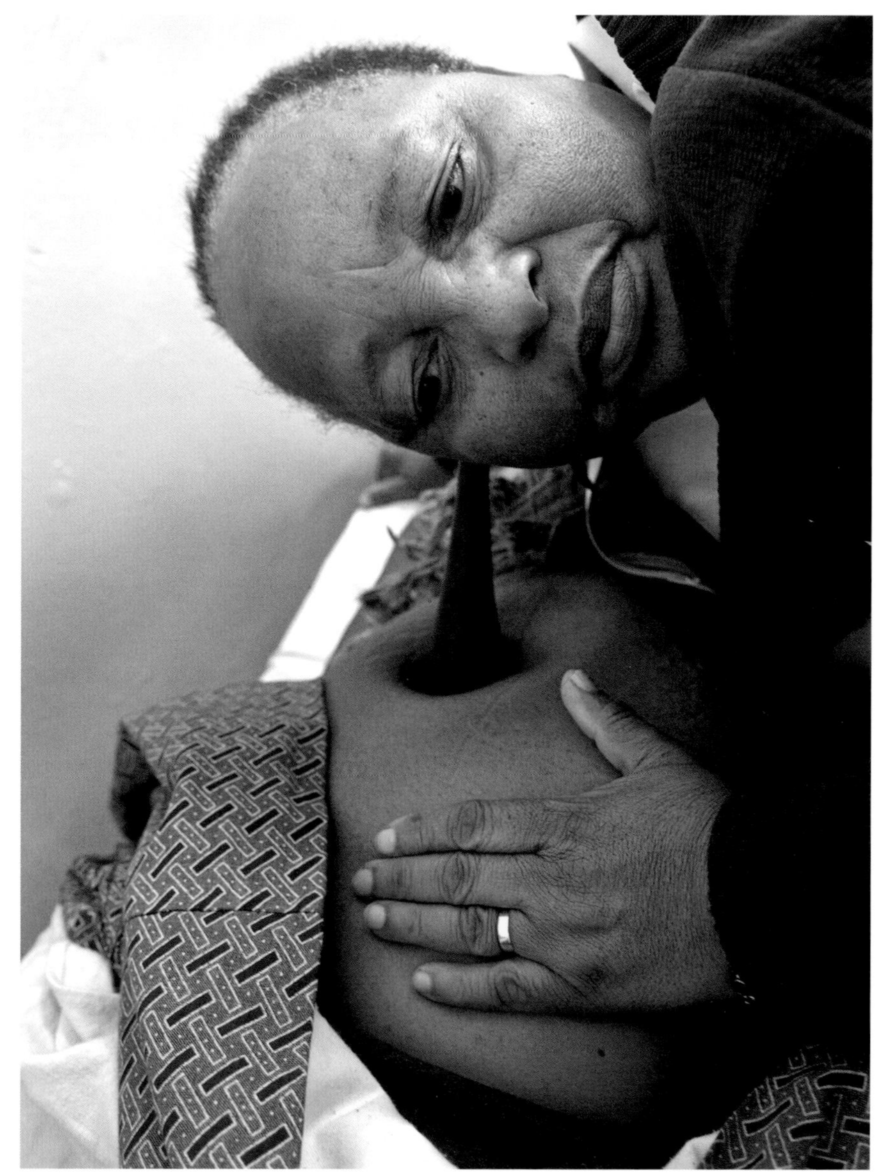

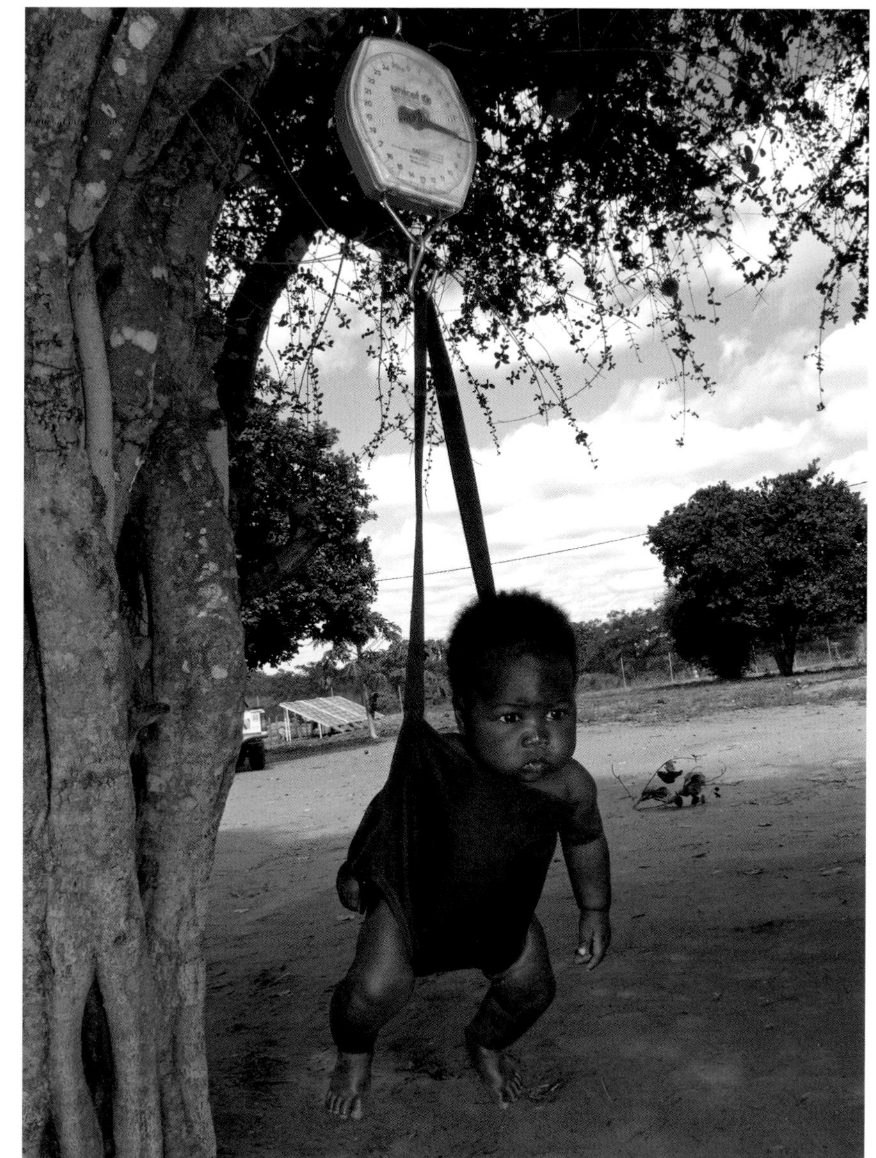

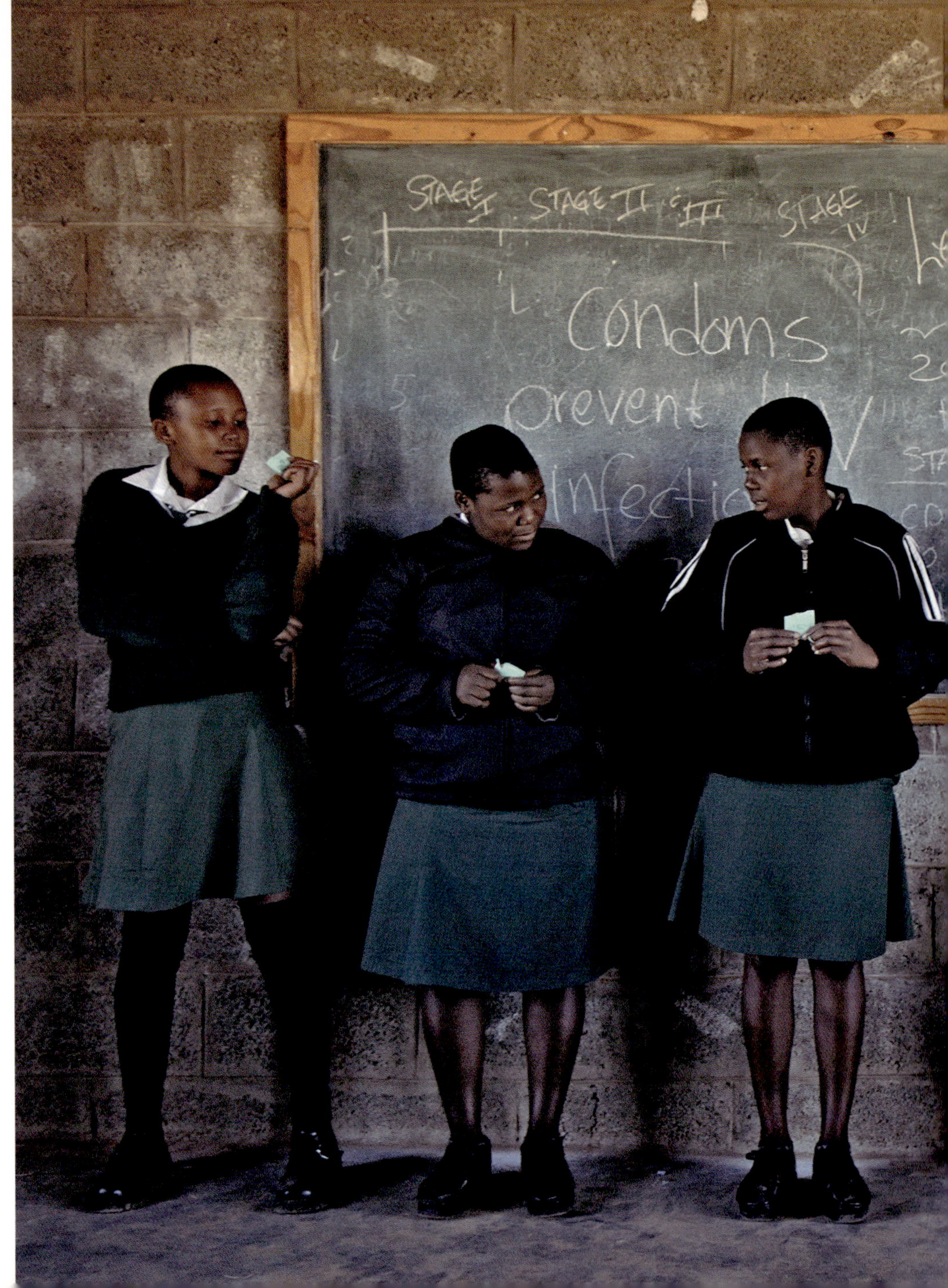
STAGE I STAGE II III STAGE
Condoms
prevent
Infection

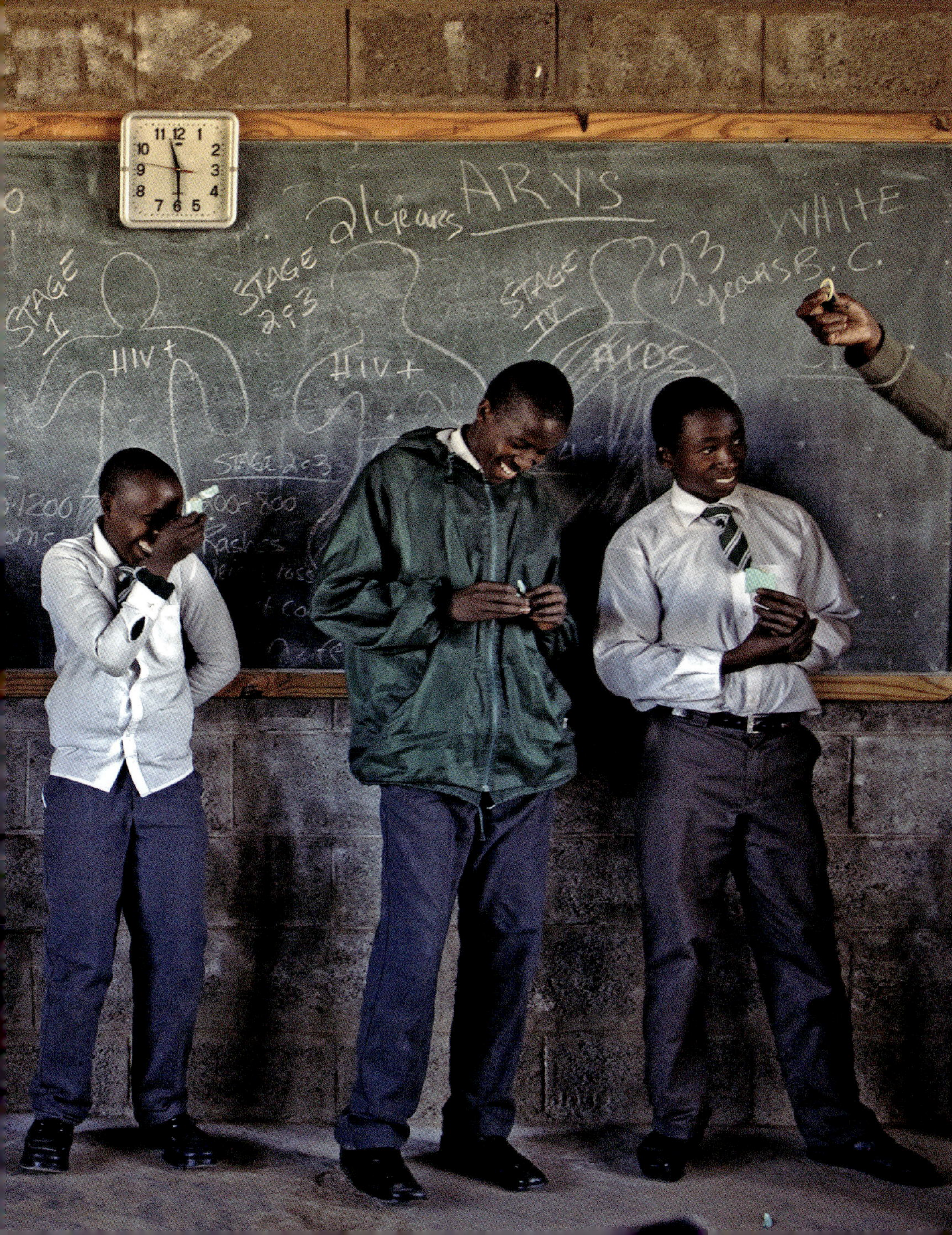

STAGE 1
HIV+
STAGE 2&3
HIV+
STAGE IV
AIDS
ARV'S
2/4 years
2&3
23 WHITE
years B.C.
STAGE 2&3
Rashes

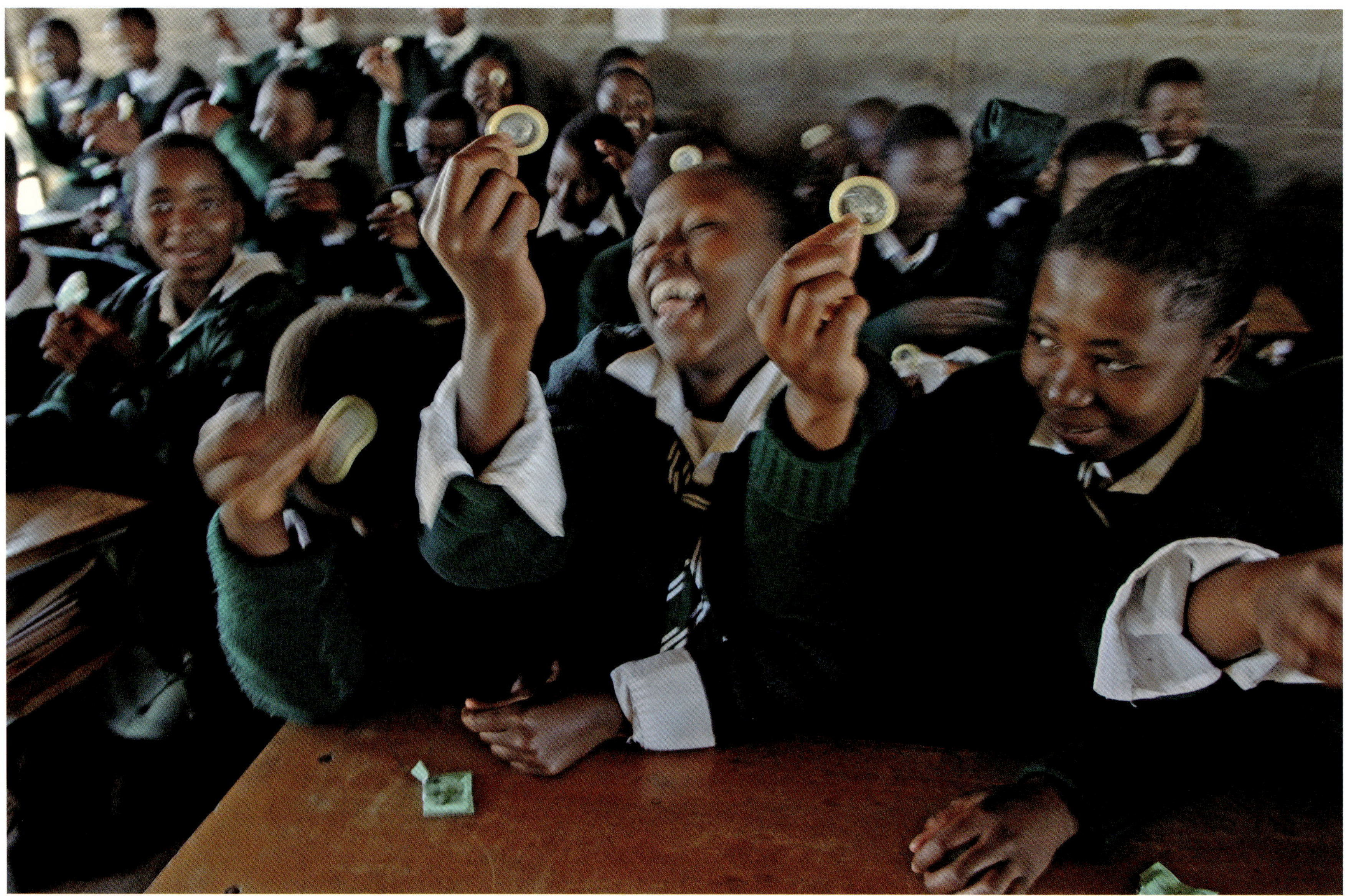

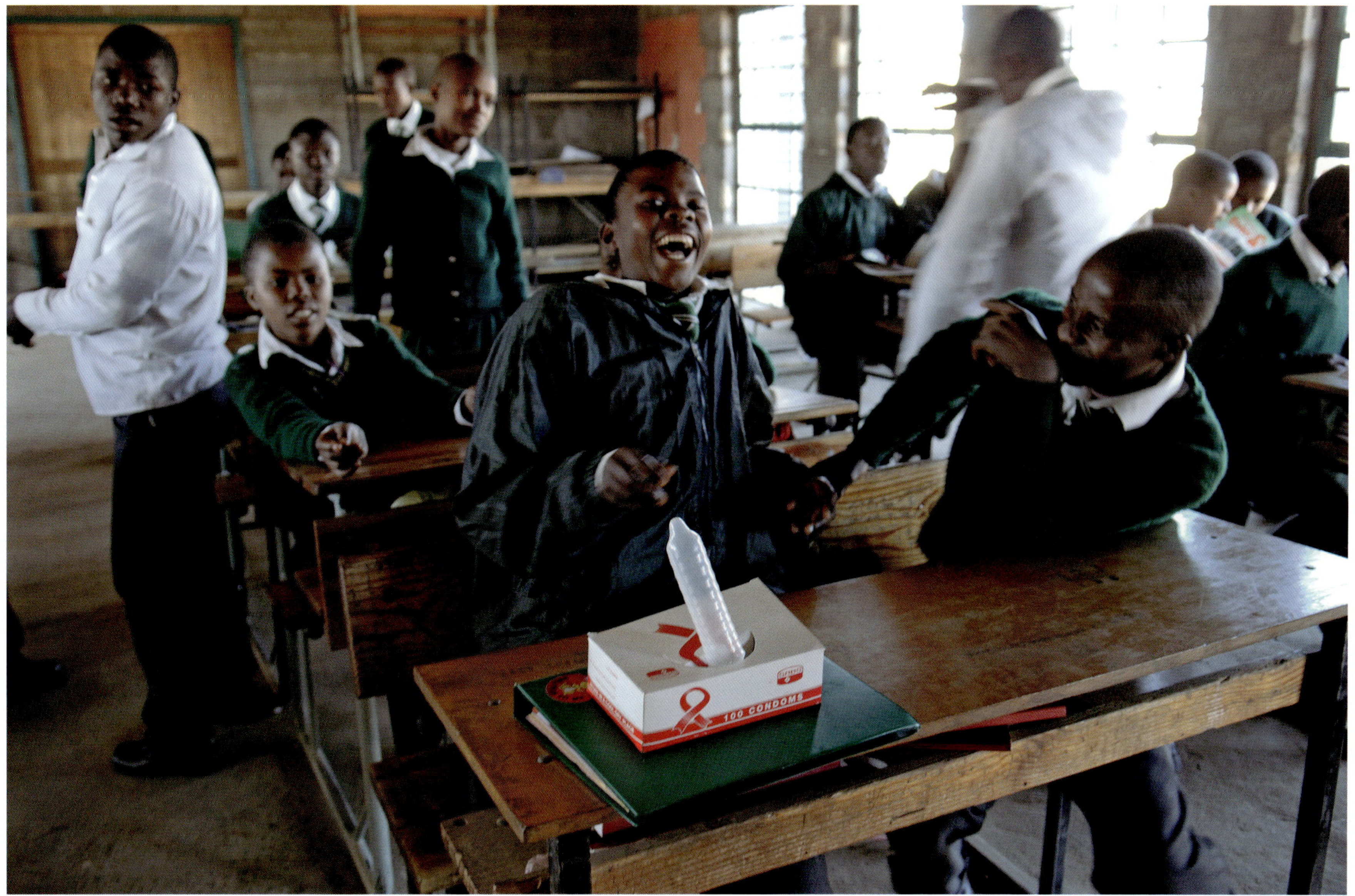

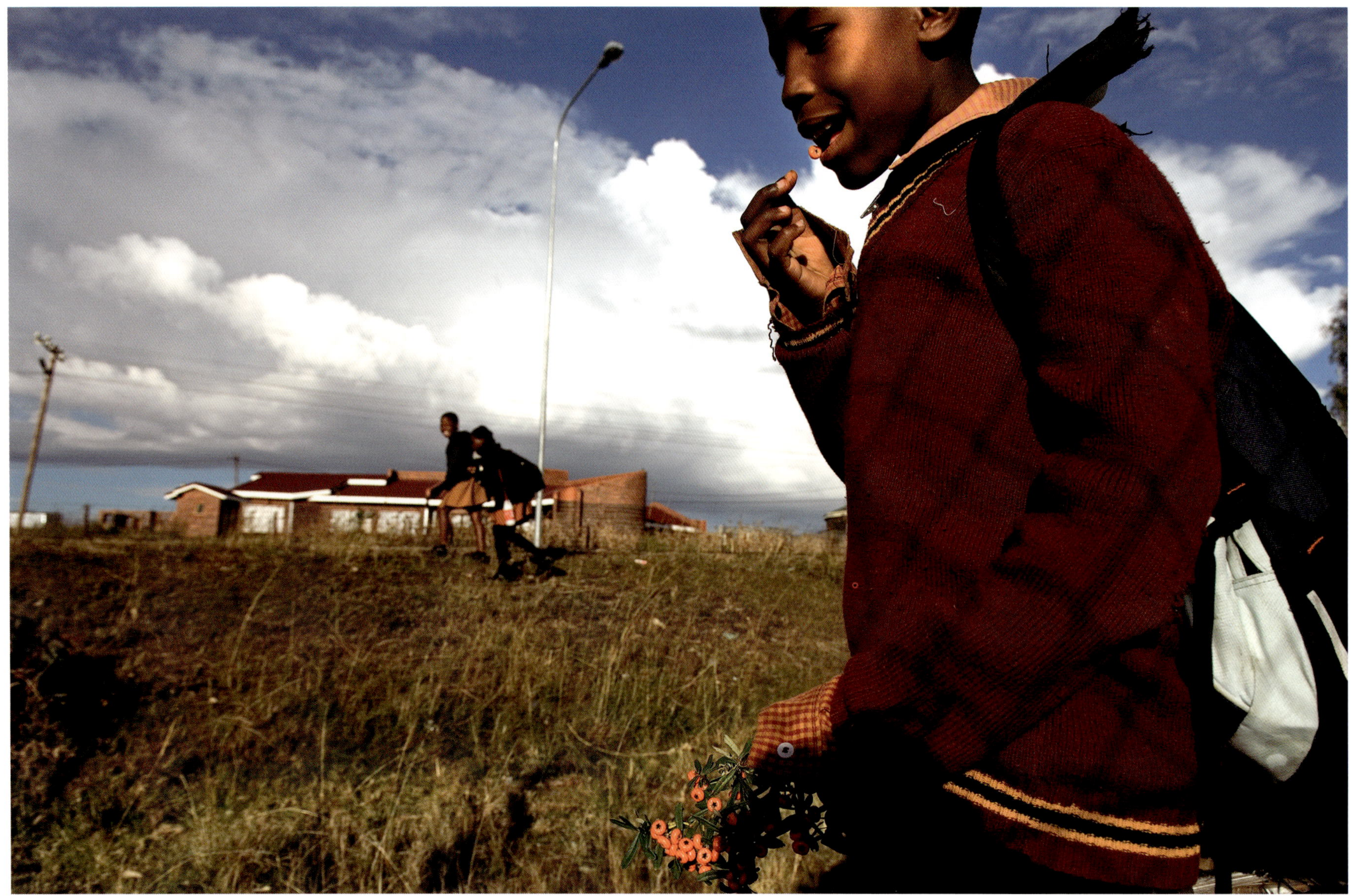

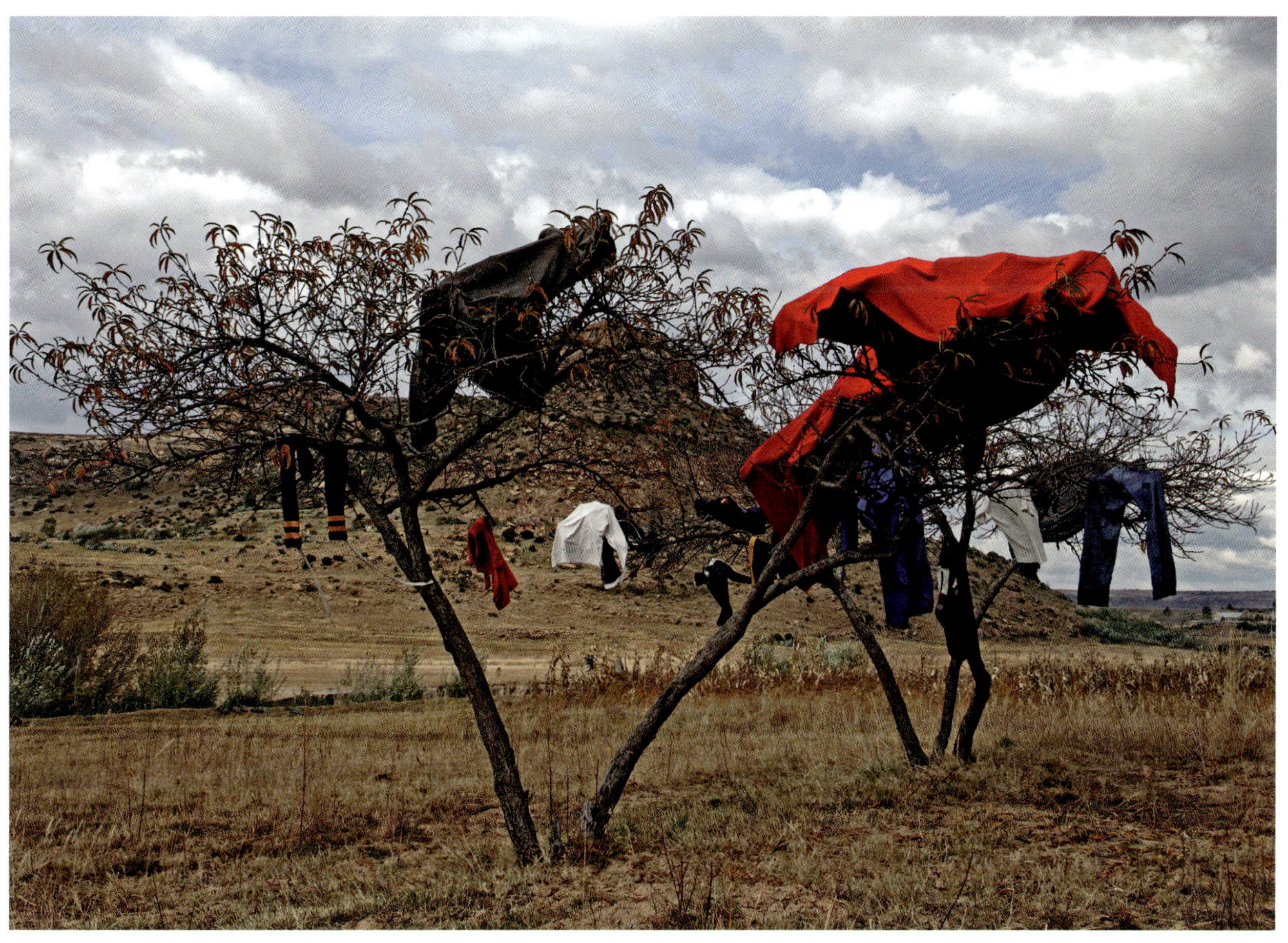

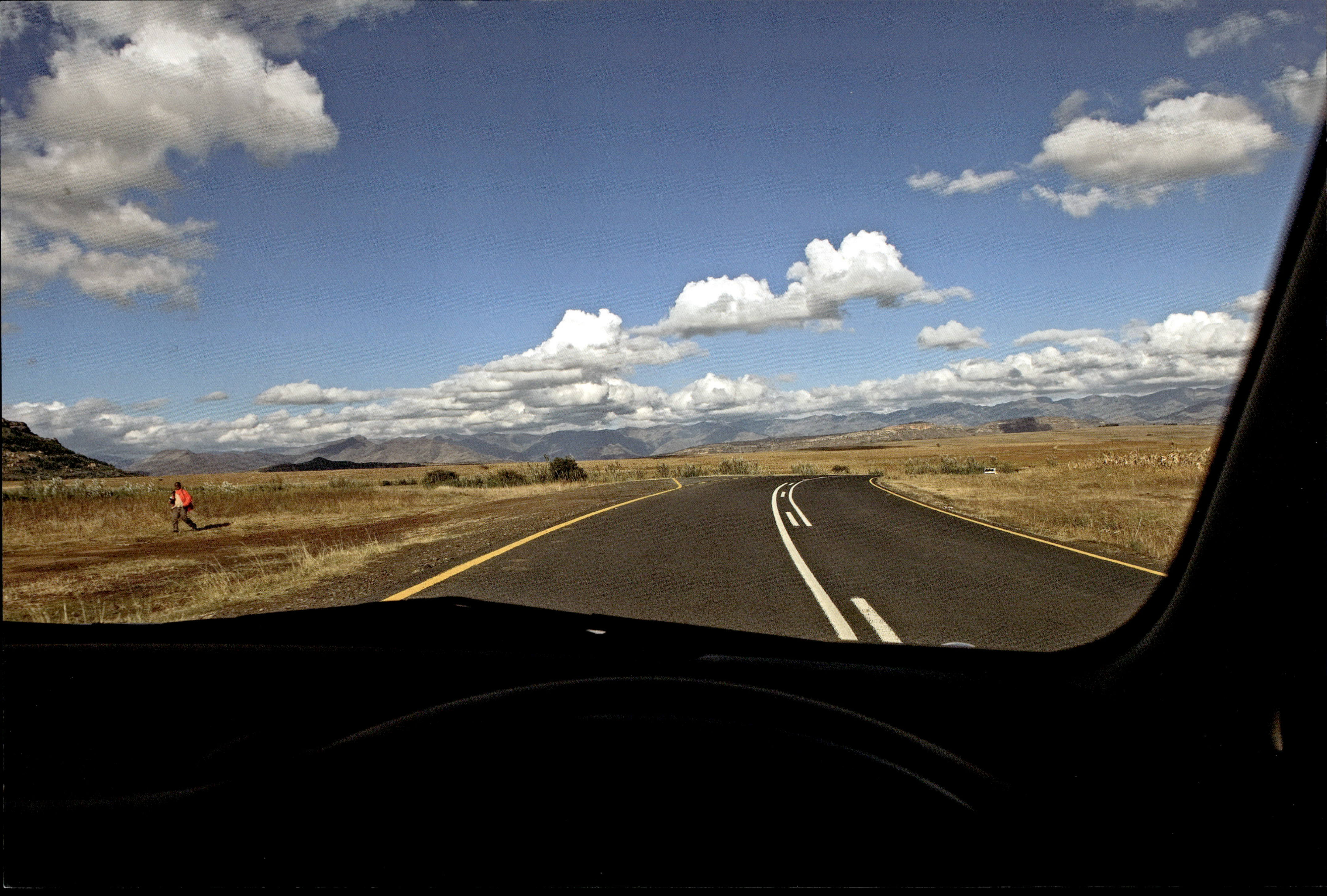

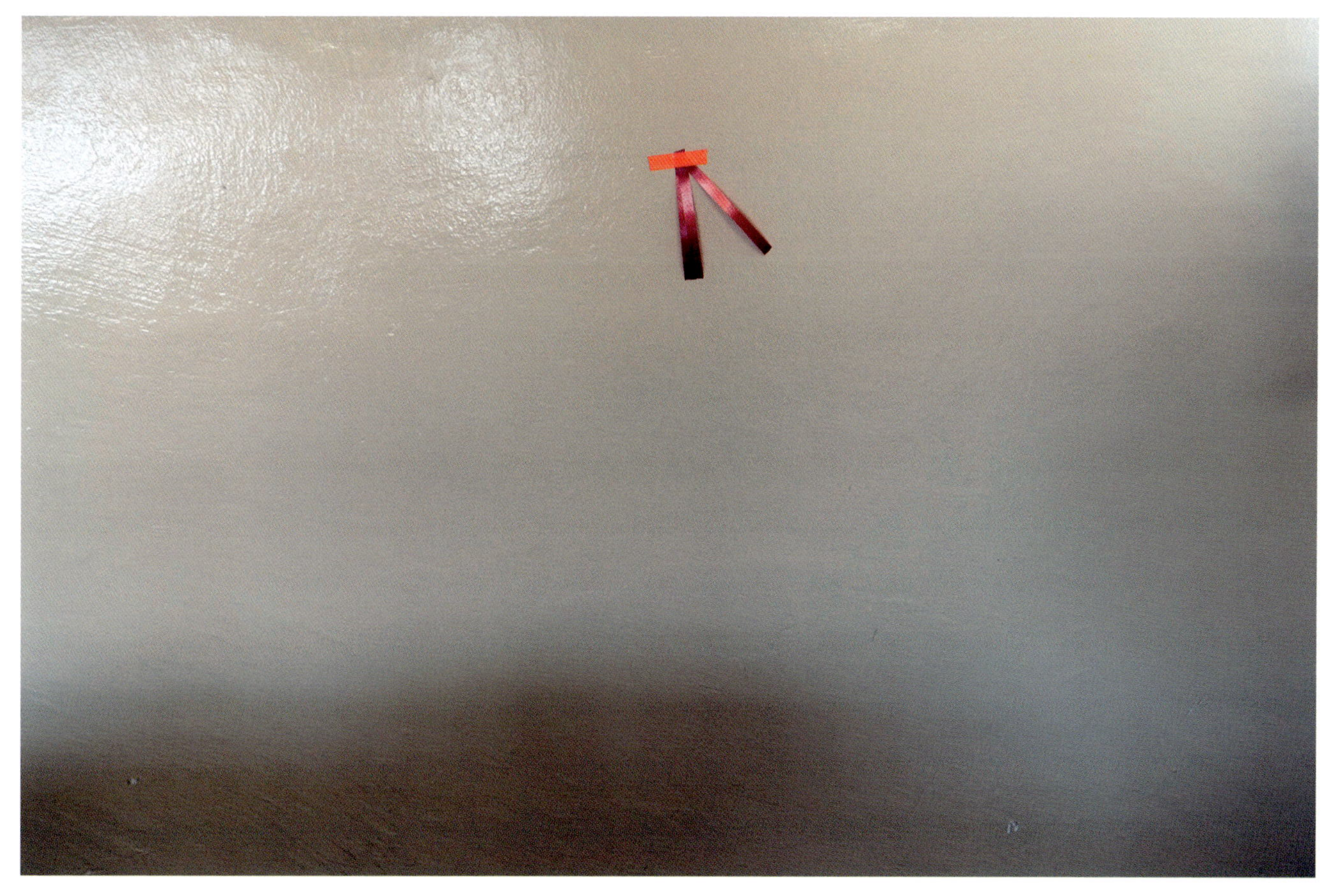

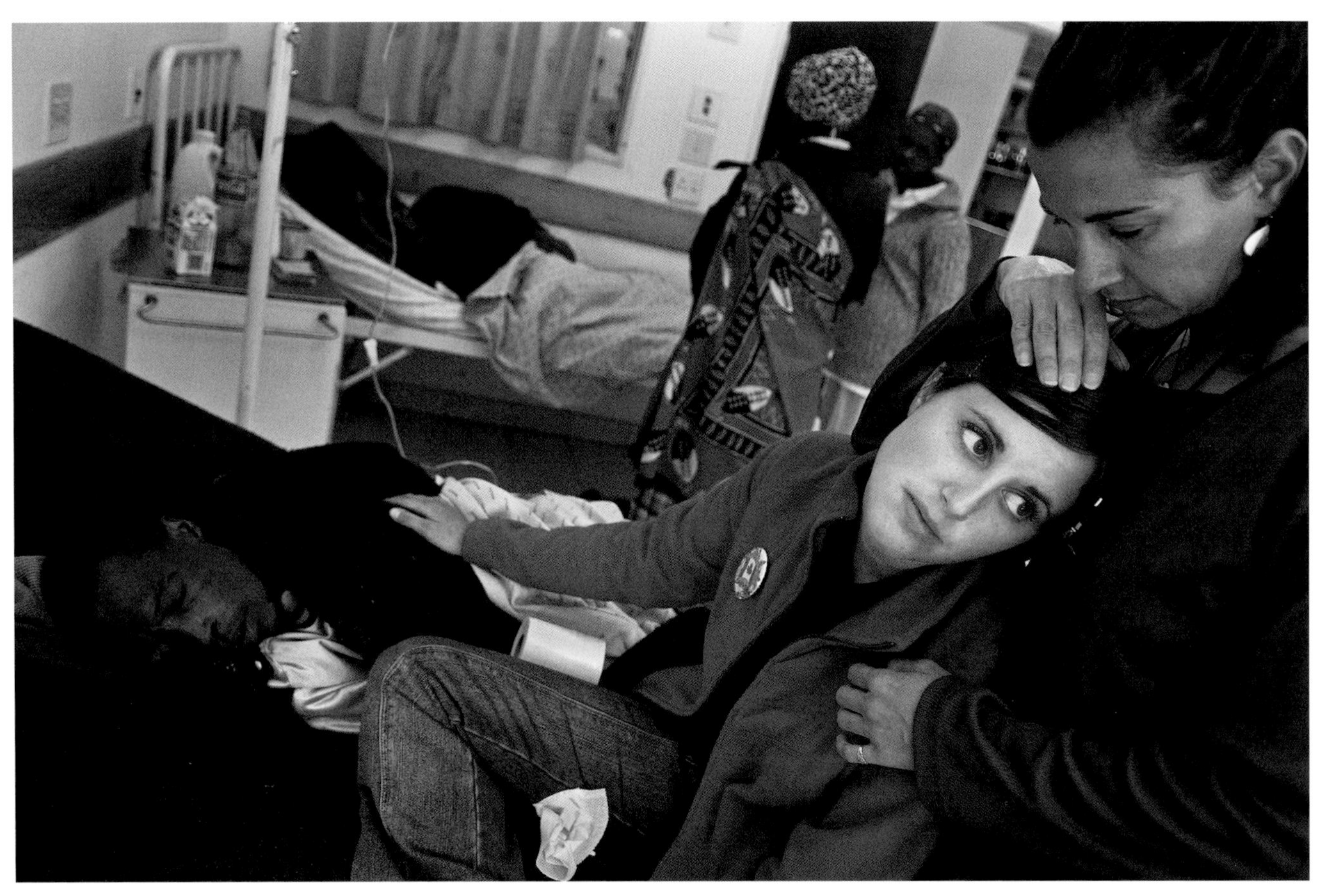

Jean Margaritis Otto, age 23
Peace Corps volunteer working with people living with AIDS, 2004–2006.

In my two years as a Peace Corps volunteer I have witnessed much that has fundamentally changed the person I am. For me, the beauty of the human spirit in Africa resides in its ability to face unimaginable tragedy with resilience, strength and love. It is in the strength of Malerato—a dying woman who struggled to bring her newborn baby for HIV testing at the hospital— and her determination to keep life going. It is the strength of Malerato's family when they found her dead body at the gate of the hospital, her newborn still cradled in her cold arms. It is the unbelievable strength that it took that family to deliver the mother's body to the mortuary, and, that same morning, to take her newly orphaned baby for HIV testing.

The resilience of the human spirit resides in the twelve-year-old orphaned girl who sells fruit day in and day out, to make sure her three younger siblings can eat. It is the compassion carried on in the children who continue to go to school, thanks to the backbreaking work of their grandmothers who just won't give up. It is the harmony in the laughter of Mamello, a young woman who volunteers her time to run a school for special-needs children in a remote village.

The African people didn't choose to live in poverty, to be stretched and pulled to the maximum, and then ravaged by the HIV pandemic. There were no other options for the young men who sacrificed an education and a future well-paying job to work as cheap labor in the mines, often under dangerous conditions, to make sure their family has something to eat. Choice isn't part of the equation when young and old women alike begin to sell their bodies for bread. What choices many do have are choices no one should ever have to make.

The choice a grandfather must make between starving all 12 of his orphaned grandchildren or adequately feeding the 7 who are not HIV-positive and will survive. The mother who must make the choice between walking 17 miles through the mountains to the nearest clinic with a two-year-old on her back while carrying another child in her arms, or leaving both at home to die without their AIDS medication.

Even with the desperation and the struggle, the beauty and warmth of the human spirit continues to radiate in Lesotho. The polyphonic sound of voices still echoes around the water tap; children still create toys out of nothing; the soccer field is always occupied by students; and grandfathers still sit around the fire telling tales of the past. Grandmothers hold grandbabies; marriages are still celebrated; and children's laughter is still contagious.

Even under the raging pandemic of the HIV virus, Africa still moves with the ancient rhythm of survival, strength and resilience. Coming from a Western nation, blessed with so many choices, I won't give up, just because it often looks like there is no other choice. We can't turn away because it looks hopeless. We have many things to learn from Africa about the human condition and the future: the most important lesson is that where love and strength exist, there is always hope.

Jean Margaritis Otto

CALL TO ACTION:
HOW YOU CAN HELP

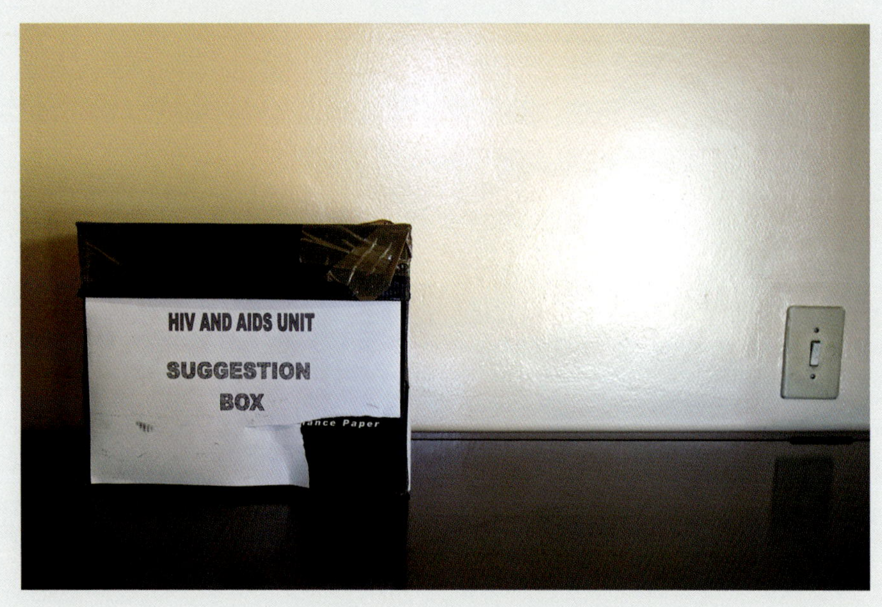

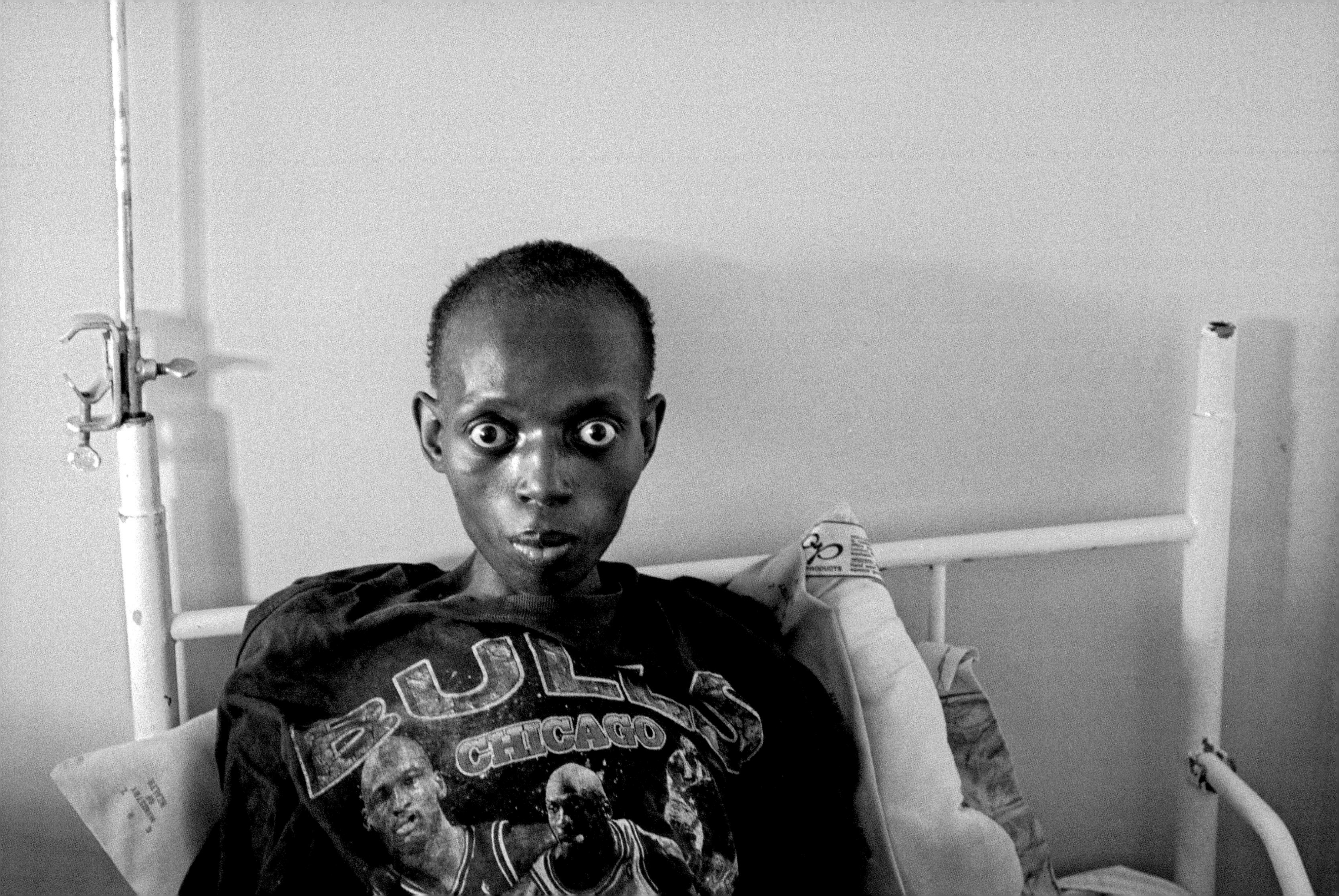

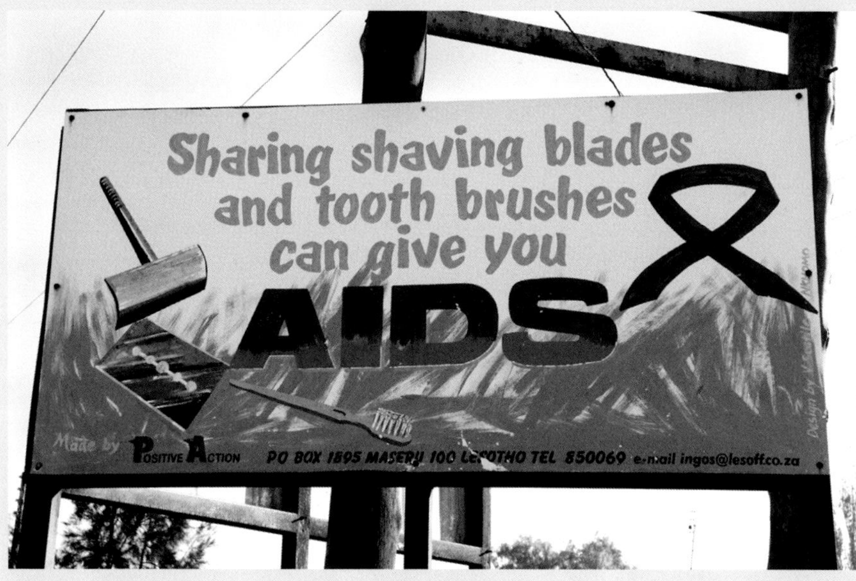

General – Members of the Global Community

The Stephen Lewis Foundation helps to ease the pain of HIV/AIDS in Africa by funding community-level projects that provide care and support to women, grandmothers, orphans and people living with AIDS. The Foundation supports over 100 projects in 14 countries in sub-Saharan Africa. They have been grateful for the support of volunteers in their Toronto office, helping with day-to-day activities. Another way to become involved is to organize events with the Stephen Lewis Foundation as the chosen beneficiary of fund-raising efforts. Visit www.stephenlewisfoundation.org to learn more. Contact: info@stephenlewisfoundation.org

Treatment Action Campaign (TAC) campaigns for treatment for people with HIV and to reduce new HIV infections. This organization's efforts have resulted in many life-saving interventions in South Africa, including the implementation of countrywide mother-to-child transmission prevention and antiretroviral treatment programs. They have offices in six provinces across South Africa, and over 14,000 volunteer members. Visit www.tac.org.za for more information. Contact: info@tac.org.za

Save the Children provides resources and social support to children affected by HIV/AIDS, by ensuring that they have access to basic services including health and education. www.savethechildren.org

Save the Children Canada is working with local organizations and communities to reduce discrimination, to provide advice and social support, to improve access to treatment and care at clinics and within communities, and to help children plan for the future after the death of a family member from HIV/AIDS. You can help in our fight against HIV/AIDS by making a gift to their Tribute program. A card will be sent to the recipient of your choice, in support of this campaign. Please visit www.savethechildren.ca for more information. Contact: volunteering@savethechildren.ca

CARE seeks a world of hope, tolerance and social justice, where poverty has been overcome and people live in dignity and security. HIV is a priority sector: projects in 15 countries work with communities to prevent new infections, facilitate care, support and give access to treatment for those infected, and build resilience to the impact of AIDS. These are complemented by humanitarian relief and development work that encompasses many other sectors (www.care.org).

Many Canadians help AIDS affected children to attend schools through **CAREConnects** (www.careconnects.ca). Organizing community events to raise funds for HIV programs is another important way to become involved with CARE's work. Visit www.care.ca to learn more about our work. Contact: info@care.ca

The Grandmothers' Campaign is a campaign of over 40 independent groups in Canada that seek to raise awareness and mobilize support for African grandmothers. The Stephen Lewis Foundation serves as a vehicle for this project to deliver support to community-level projects in Africa. Visit www.stephenlewisfoundation.org for more information. Contact: info@stephenlewisfoundation.org

Engineers Without Borders (EWB) aims to promote human development and strives to drive change in Canada and in developing communities. Volunteers promote human development in some of the world's most impoverished communities. You can become involved in EWB in a number of ways ranging from donations, becoming a member, joining a chapter, volunteering overseas, running a workplace campaign and/or inviting EWB to your high school classroom. Please visit www.ewb.ca for more information. Contact: info@ewb.ca

African Medical and Research Foundation (AMREF)'s mission is to improve the health of disadvantaged people in Africa as a means to escape poverty and improve quality of life. Their mission determines that they work in specific priority intervention areas. With 35 HIV/AIDS/TB related projects across Africa, AMREF works at the front line of the campaign to attain universal access to HIV/AIDS and TB prevention, care, treatment and impact mitigation. AMREF has offices in Europe, USA and Canada. These offices primarily raise funds for their programs in Africa. For more information, please visit www.amref.org

World Vision is a Christian humanitarian advocacy, relief and development organization active in more than 90 countries around the world, providing help to more than 85 million people each year in the areas of emergency relief, education, health care, economic development and the promotion of justice. Log on to www.wvi.org for more information on how to get involved. Contact: info@world-vision.org

Foster Parents Plan is one of the world's largest international, child-centered development organizations. They work in 45 developing countries where, worldwide, their long-term community programs benefit 1.3 million children and impact the lives of 13 million people. There are a number of different ways to get involved with FPP including corporate partnerships, fundraising, child sponsorship, the youth advisory council and volunteering. Please visit www.plancanada.ca for more information. Contact: info@fosterparentsplan.ca

Saltspring Organization for Life Improvement and Development (SOLID) is a nonprofit society dedicated to support and empower HIV/AIDS affected families in sub-Saharan Africa. As part of SOLID, the **Phelisanong Disabled Group** is a community-based organization designed to help orphans, people who are suffering from physical or mental disabilities, and those with HIV. It was begun by its current director, Mamello Lehlotha, in 2001 and has since grown to include several departments, including a preschool, a sewing school, HIV/AIDS support groups (one for adults and one for young people), a craft-making group, and agriculture. The project seeks ultimately to become a self-sustaining community where the various needs of the above-mentioned groups can be met. Please visit www.solidsaltspring.com for more information. To correspond directly: Phelisanong, Pitseng Box 480, Leribe 300 Lesotho. Contact: info@solidsaltspring.com

The **Mother of Mercy Hospice** was established in 1992 by Sister Leonia Komas, a Polish nun and registered nurse, to provide care for terminally ill AIDS patients in the community of Chilanga, approximately 16 km south of Lusaka, Zambia. Over the last decade, Mother of Mercy has expanded, responding to the growing needs of individual adults, families, and children in the local community who are impacted by HIV/AIDS. The organization reaches out into the community to identify households in need. The most common support needed is medical care and palliative support of AIDS patients, food, and schooling for children. The core of Mother of Mercy is a

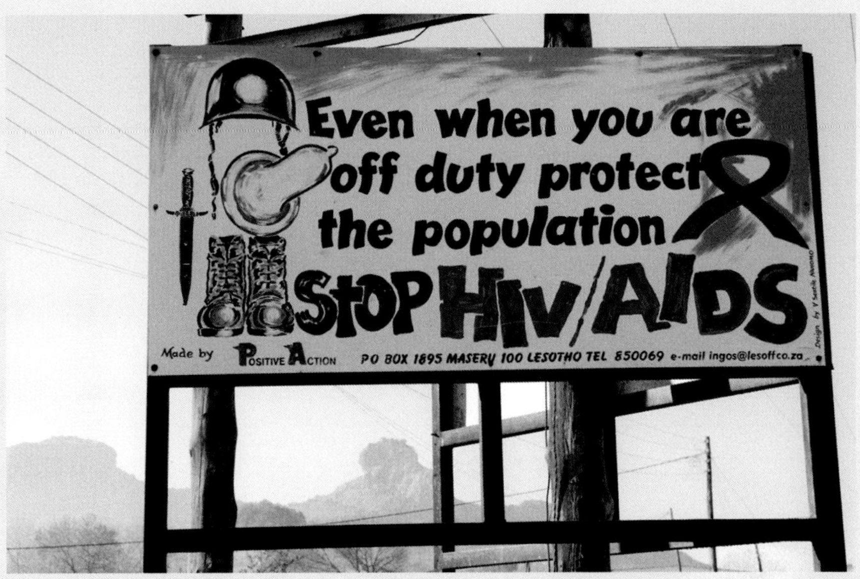

home-based care program, though additional assistance is provided through a 22-bed inpatient hospice, an outpatient clinic, and a community school. Sister Leonia Komas, P.O. Box 350080, Chilanga, Zambia – Tel.: +260 1 278 539 – Mobile: +260 96 744 074 Contact: hospicel@zamnet.zm

The **Power of Love Foundation** is a U.S. nonprofit that was founded in 2002 to develop community responses to the AIDS crisis in Africa. Their mission is to turn back the tide of the global AIDS epidemic through innovative community responses that increase the effectiveness of prevention and care efforts. Their vision: A world where the AIDS epidemic is in continuous retreat and people living with HIV have access to loving care and treatment in an environment free of stigma and discrimination. The foundation funds programs in Kenya and Zambia independently. They found two significant problems that moved them to action: The fight against the AIDS epidemic was being fought in the communities, but little funding was going there. Second, what little funding was going to community AIDS relief organizations was most often needed to fulfill immediate on-the-ground requirements. The foundation believes that by utilizing technology and business processes more funding could be attracted to communities. Go to www.poweroflove.org for more information. Contact: info@poweroflove.org

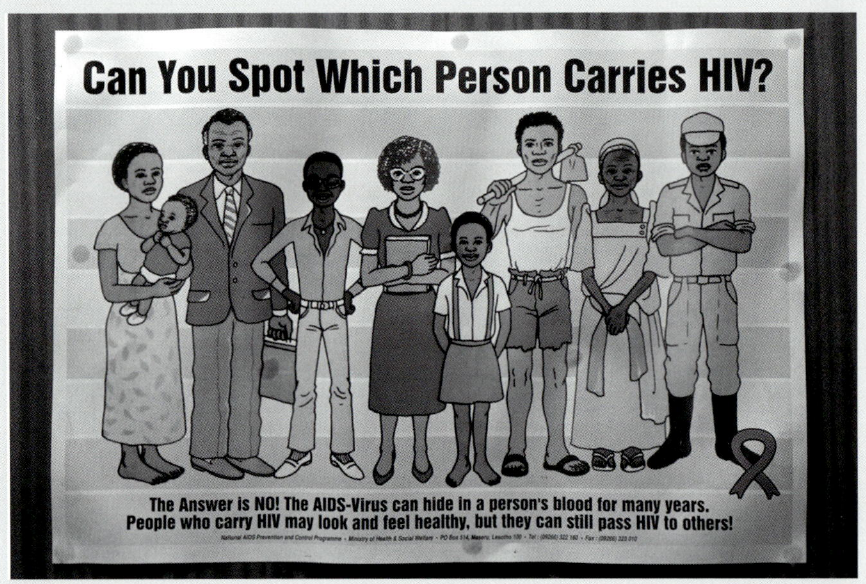

Businesses

The **Global Fund to Fight AIDS, Tuberculosis and Malaria** was created to finance a dramatic turn-around in the fight against AIDS, tuberculosis and malaria. The Global Fund attracts, manages and disburses resources in a number of ways, including ARV treatment programs, counseling and testing services for HIV prevention, and providing medical treatment, education and community care for AIDS orphans. Please visit www.theglobalfund.org for more information on how you can contribute. Contact: info@theglobalfund.org

The **Southern African AIDS Trust** (SAT) is a regional organization aiming to increase the HIV and AIDS competence of communities in southern Africa. SAT strives to be a leader in capacity building of CBOs and NGOs. SAT operates in four different areas: Capacity development partnerships with regional organizations; regional skills training and lessons sharing; networks; and research and documentation strategy and publications. Contributions to this program are greatly appreciated. Please visit www.satregional.org for more information. Contact: info@satregional.org

Educators

AVERT is an international HIV and AIDS organization that has a number of overseas projects, helping with the response to HIV/AIDS in countries where there is a particularly high rate of infection, such as South Africa, or where there is a rapidly increasing rate of infection such as in India. Developed over a number of years, AVERT.org now has a wide range of information that includes factual information about HIV/AIDS, specific areas for people to visit for more information, and a choice of educational resources including downloadable booklets and quizzes. Please visit www.avert.org for more information about AVERT and/or to contribute. Contact: info@avert.org

Centre for HIV/AIDS Networking (HIVAN) strives to enhance the quality of HIV/AIDS prevention, care and treatment in both the formal and informal public health systems by connecting multidisciplinary scholarship with the immediate needs and problems of health-care providers, civil-society organizations, and communities. At the heart of HIVAN—and serving as its driving intellectual and strategic force—is a team of biomedical, social and behavioral scientists dedicated to initiating and undertaking multi-disciplinary research programs. Please visit www.hivan.org.za for more information. Contact: admin@hivan.org.za

Tsepong Counselling Centre, Sebaboleng/Maseru, Lesotho, was established in 2001 to raise HIV/AIDS awareness, to provide counseling services, to support orphans and vulnerable children, and to empower communities through knowledge and home-based care. The center focuses on counseling and AIDS prevention work. They currently run four village-level orphan support groups and regularly facilitate HIV/AIDS prevention and training nationwide. They also support 15 orphans with food, home visits and counseling. They provide skills training for children, and training for caregivers and village support groups in orphan issues, home-based care, and counseling skills. Contact: tsepongcc@leo.co.ls

OHAfrica is a joint initiative of the Ontario Hospital Association and The Change Foundation, who are working in close partnership with the Government of Lesotho. OHAfrica came into being in response to the challenge made to Ontario hospitals by Stephen Lewis, the UN Secretary General's Special Envoy for HIV/AIDS in Africa, to play a leadership role in helping to treat and prevent the spread of HIV/AIDS in Africa. At Mr. Lewis's recommendation, the southern African country of Lesotho was chosen as the focus of the project. OHAfrica supports the implementation of the newly introduced antiretroviral (ARV) drug therapy program for people living with HIV/AIDS in Lesotho. Visit www.ohafrica.ca for more information. Contact: info@oha.com

Médecins Sans Frontières (MSF) is the world's leading international humanitarian aid organization providing independent emergency medical assistance to populations in danger in over 70 countries. In MSF field projects, international volunteers work alongside national staff in medical, paramedical, logistical and administrative positions. In 2006, MSF currently treats over 60,000 adults and children living with HIV/AIDS in 29 countries. Visit www.msf.org for more information.

Association of Nurses in AIDS Care (ANAC) is composed of a dedicated group of nurses, healthcare professionals and others who are committed to HIV/AIDS nursing. With a highly regarded peer-reviewed journal, and an Annual Conference featuring national and international speakers and educational and scientific sessions on the latest developments in HIV nursing, ANAC is meeting the needs of nurses in HIV/AIDS care, research, prevention and policy. Please visit www.anac-net.org to learn more about becoming a member. Contact: anac@anacnet.org

The primary purpose of the **International Association of Physicians in AIDS Care** (IAPAC) is to craft and implement global educational and advocacy strategies to improve the quality of care provided to all people living with HIV/AIDS. IAPAC's strength is firmly rooted in the belief that the most effective and creative solutions to ongoing issues of access to HIV treatment evolve from within the association's membership. IAPAC's membership consists of a growing network of physicians and allied healthcare professionals from over 100 countries. Please visit www.iapac.org for more information. Contact: iapac@iapac.org

Helping AIDS in Resource-Poor Countries (HARPA) seeks to enable visits by HIV medical specialists from resource-rich areas to HIV projects in resource-poor areas. Similarly, HARPA also seeks to enable visiting training scholarships for HIV medical providers from resource-poor areas to visit resource-rich areas for HIV medical training. HARPA also aims to provide a library of clinical and educational materials and a directory of organizations worldwide who are involved in the provision of HIV medical care and education in resource-poor areas through our website. HARPA gladly accepts contributions in the form of volunteers and/or donations. Please visit http://www.harpa.org for more information. Contact: douglui@harpa.org

TakingITGlobal.org (TIG) is an online community led by youth and empowered by technology that connects youth to find inspiration, access information, get involved, and take action in their local and global communities. There are many ways to get involved with TIG including volunteering, internships, co-ops and work placements. Please visit www.takingit-global.org for more information. Contact: info@takingitglobal.org

Youth Challenge International builds skills, experience and confidence of young people by involving them in substantive overseas international development projects in partnership with local youth-serving organizations. Volunteers participate in projects taking place in South and Central America, the South Pacific and Africa. Besides working alongside local youth to address the issues they face, program contribution funds raised by the volunteers are distributed among the local organizations in the host country to support their efforts addressing development issues in their own country. Please visit www.yci.org for more information. Contact: generalinfo@yci.org

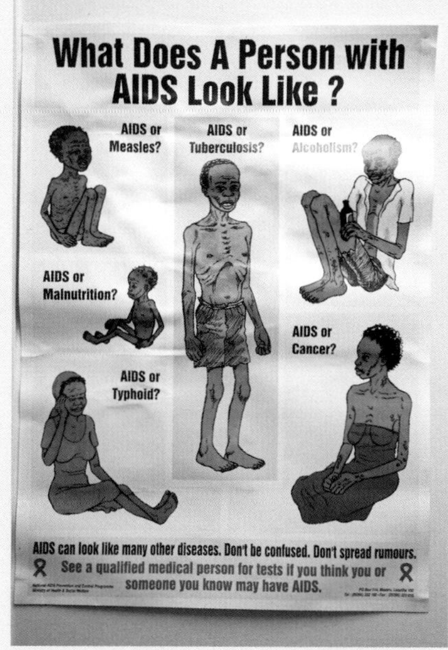

World University Service of Canada (WUSC) is a network of individuals and post-secondary institutions aiming to foster human development and global understanding through education and training. Through WUSC you can help build a more equitable world by working, volunteering or learning in a developing country. From two weeks to two years, we offer experiences in international development for people that range from undergraduate students to mid-career experts to retirees. Please visit www.wusc.ca for more information. Contact: wusc@wusc.ca

AIDS: Picture Change is a traveling photo exhibition and youth campaign supported by the Canadian Coalition on HIV/AIDS and Youth in Africa that aims to educate and engage youth in the global struggle against HIV/AIDS. There are many creative ways to become involved in this project by taking action in your own community and documenting your experiences on the AIDS: Picture Change website. Please visit www.picturechange.ca for more information. Contact: info@picturechange.ca

Athletes

Right to Play is an international humanitarian organization using sport and play as tools for the development of children and youth in the most disadvantaged areas of the world. Volunteers typically have formal education and experience in one or more of the following areas: sport, recreation or physical education; child development; community development; international development; adult education; training of trainers or coaches; education and curriculum development; public health promotion; HIV/AIDS awareness; social work; working with people with disabilities; and communications or public relations. Please visit www.righttoplay.com for more information. Contact: recruitment@righttoplay.com

Community-based Organizations

ALL OUT Africa is based in Swaziland and implements progressive volunteer projects in South Africa, Mozambique and Swaziland. Our mission is to understand and improve the welfare of people and wildlife in Africa through research, volunteer projects and responsible tourism. Volunteer projects focus on social issues surrounding HIV and AIDS in Swaziland and South Africa as well as conservation. Volunteers are posted at daycare centers for orphaned and vulnerable children (OVCs), are involved in education, feeding, life skills training, agriculture, and basic care and attention giving. Please visit www.all-out.org for more information. Contact: kim@all-out.org or rols@all-out.org

The **Terrence Higgins Trust** (THT) is the leading HIV and AIDS charity in the UK and the largest in Europe. The objectives of THT are to reduce the spread of HIV and STIs, to promote good sexual health, to provide services that improve the health and quality of life of those affected, and to campaign for greater public understanding of the personal, social and medical impact of HIV and sexual ill health. Volunteers help in a number of ways including community support, helpline and administration. Please visit www.tht.org.uk for more information. Contact: info@tht.org.uk

Casey House is a hospice providing compassionate palliative and supportive care for people with HIV/AIDS in Toronto, Canada. Volunteers contribute many thousands of hours of skilled, passionate and compassionate work that enables Casey House to serve more people with HIV/AIDS. Some of the services provided by volunteers are administrative support, assistance with resident care and comfort, educational talks and training, gardening and plant care, hairdressing, housekeeping, kitchen help and meal service, library services, newsletter production and reception coverage. Visit www.caseyhouse.com or contact: info@caseyhouse.on.ca

San Francisco AIDS Foundation provides direct services to thousands of people living with or at risk for HIV/AIDS, supplies information about HIV treatment and related issues, promotes HIV prevention and awareness in the community, and advocates for sound HIV/AIDS policies at all levels of government. From staffing the hotline to supporting fundraising efforts, from licking stamps to stuffing envelopes, volunteers are a critical component of day-to-day work. Please visit www.sfaf.org for more information. Contact: feedback@sfaf.org

New York Harm Reduction Educators, Inc. (NYHRE) was formed to prevent the spread of AIDS by offering harm-reduction services. NYHRE takes a harm reduction approach by promoting safer injecting and safer sex practices and by helping participants gain access to medical and social services. People can become involved in NYHRE in a number of ways ranging from service delivery staff, management, volunteers and clients. Please visit www.nyhre.org for more information.

The **Mario Mieli Association for Homosexual Culture** is a nonprofit organization established in 1984 to promote and protect the rights of gay, lesbian, bisexual and transsexual people. Main activities include: welcome, orientation and information reception services; legal and medical assistance; a psychological advice bureau; social and medical assistance to HIV-positive people; education efforts for high school students regarding diversity, increased awareness regarding sexual behavior and HIV prevention; a mobile health unit for the prevention of HIV and STDs; counseling services and assistance to accompany HIV testing in San Giovanni Hospital, Rome; and support groups for HIV-positive people. Visit www.mariomieli.org for more information. Contact info@mariomieli.org

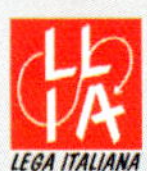

The **Italian League for the Fight Against Aids** (LILA) is a nonprofit organization founded in 1987 that operates at a national level through its local branches. It is a federation composed of associations and groups of seropositive and seronegative volunteers and professionals. At the national level it is comprised of different service areas, also conducting research on therapies, risk behaviors, assistance and prevention. In addition, the national offices aim at influencing the development of social and sanitary policies, as well as offering support to local branches operating at regional, provincial and community levels. LILA promotes and defends the rights of people to health; it is committed to the principles of solidarity, and it fights violations of human and civil rights of people living with HIV and AIDS through the organization of psychological and social integration services. LILA collaborates with other Italian and European NGOs, as well as important national institutions. Visit www.lila.it for more information. Contact lila@lila.it

Biography

Steve Simon was born in Montreal in 1960. He has been passionate about documenting life through photography since he began taking photographs at age 12 in his home city of Montreal.

He studied Journalism/Communications at Concordia University and photography at the Dawson Institute Of Photography, both in Montreal. He later taught photojournalism at Loyalist College before moving to New York City to concentrate on documentary photography.

He has had solo shows in New York, Buenos Aires, Toronto and Montreal, and his work has been featured three times at the Visa Pour L'Image Photography Festival in Perpignan, France. His work is in the permanent collections of The George Eastman House, the Houston Museum of Fine Arts and the Comune di Verona. Recent work has been published in *Mother Jones*, *The New York Times Magazine*, *Life*, *Colors*, *GEO*, *Le Monde*, *Walrus* and *Harpers*.

Simon has received numerous international awards including the Global Health Council Photography Award for his work on AIDS in Africa, the Canadian Newspaper Photographer of the Year, the National Press Photographers Association Picture of the Year, an Alfred Eisenstaedt Magazine Photography Award, the Art Director's Club of New York Award, the Canadian Association of Journalists Photojournalism Award and the Canadian Press News Picture of the Year. He has participated as a guest lecturer and workshop leader at various photojournalism and arts events in Canada, the United States, and Argentina.

He has three previously published books: *The Republicans*, on the 2004 Republican Convention in New York City, published by Charta; *Healing Waters*, which documents the healing powers of a small lake in Alberta; and *Empty Sky: The Pilgrimage to Ground Zero*, an excerpt of which was included in Time-Life's book *The American Spirit*, forward by George W. Bush.

He is based in New York City.

To see more, please visit www.stevesimonphoto.com

Captions

p. 2 Chief Alina Seqhibolla, 95, of Ha Majara in Lesotho, has 8 children, 28 grandchildren and 17 great-grandchildren. For many, grandmothers have become the heart of the response to the HIV/AIDS epidemic as the guardians of children who represent the future and hope of Africa.

p. 8 An orphaned boy at Phelisanong, a community-based project to rehabilitate, educate and train disabled children and youth. They provide HIV education, support groups and outreach for orphans and other vulnerable children. See Call To Action.

p. 9 *Top:* Pheello Lintle, three hours old at the Military Hospital in Lesotho.
Bottom: Steve Simon with Alex Sekikila (1963–2006).

p. 10 The AIDS symbol on a hill near Maseru, Lesotho, is one of many AIDS ribbons painted by local support groups on nearby mountains as part of ongoing HIV awareness campaigns.

p. 11 Chief Joseph Tseea from the village of Haramoabi, teacher and Red Cross volunteer.

p. 12 Schoolgirls cross the road near the town of Hlotse, Lesotho. In Africa, a young person is infected with HIV every 14 seconds. Young people (increasingly young women) account for nearly half of the new cases of HIV infection worldwide.

p. 13 A young man rides horseback just outside of Teyateyaneng, Lesotho. For many in Lesotho, ranked by the United Nations as one of the poorest countries in the world, there is no escape from poverty.

p. 14 Bennett Nkokana, 30, and Adellina Kholu, 25, sit and talk by the side of the road on the outskirts of Holtse, Lesotho.

p. 15 This is the view from the top of the hill in the village of Ha Majara in Lesotho. Small-scale farming and other income-generating activities are part of comprehensive HIV/AIDS prevention and treatment programs. Economy-building programs focus on women's empowerment and rights.

p. 16 The body of Woyneshet Danieal, who died of AIDS at 35, is carried to the cemetery near Harare, Ethiopia. The HIV epidemic has evolved in Ethiopia from two reported AIDS cases in 1986 to a cumulative total of 147,000 by mid-2003.

p. 17 Grandmother Maputse Moriti, 79, is a cook for Phelisanong, a community-based project to rehabilitate, educate and train disabled children and youth. They provide HIV education, support groups and outreach for orphans and other vulnerable children. She has 28 grandchildren.

p. 18 At a cemetery near Harare, Ethiopia, Nega Wondimu chips away at what will eventually become a headstone. Ethiopia is one of the countries more severely affected by HIV/AIDS. The number of people currently living with HIV/AIDS in Ethiopia is estimated to be 1.5 million. The HIV prevalence in rural areas is 2.3%, as opposed to a prevalence of 13.2% in urban areas.

p. 19 A small church in Maputsoe, Lesotho, led by Pastor Moses Marshall.

pp. 20-21 The city market in Maseru, Lesotho, is busy in the late afternoon. Based on indicators of poverty, human resources and economic diversification, Lesotho is ranked 145 out of 177 countries on the United Nations Development Program.

p. 22 Two bibles at a small church in Maputsoe, Lesotho, led by Pastor Moses Marshall.

p. 23 Gilda Manuel Mate with son Vasco Moises and daughter Dercia Moises at her kitchen table. She is HIV-positive and a spokesperson in the fight against AIDS. She lives in Fidel Castro Village, Mabote, Mozambique.

p. 24 Science and Wonders Ministries in Maputsoe, Lesotho, is lead by Pastor Diapuleng Angela Sekamane.

p. 25 Mathabisang Leputla gives testimony about her life, including her HIV-positive status, in front of the congregation at a church in Maputsoe, Lesotho. She is now an AIDS educator encouraging people to get tested and take care of themselves.

p. 26 A man and women lit by candlelight at a bar in Mabote, Mozambique. A breakdown of estimated infection rates by province shows that central provinces in Mozambique are the most affected by the HIV virus. In the Inhambane province, where this photograph was taken, 18% of adults are thought to be HIV-positive.

p. 27 Young men photographed outside the Ha Sekekete Hotel bar in Maputsoe, Lesotho, near the South African border. One challenge AIDS-prevention educators face is changing men's attitudes toward gender and promoting communication between men and women regarding condom use.

p. 28 Young men line up at the bar in Mabote, Mozambique. UNAIDS estimates that people under 25 years old account for half of all new HIV infections.

p. 29 A dance floor, photographed at a bar in Vilanculos, Mozambique. Around 59% of all adults living with HIV in sub-Saharan Africa are women.

p. 30 Prostitutes frequent many bars in Addis Ababa, Ethiopia. They are often paid extra to have sex without a condom, which contributes to the high rate of HIV transmission. In some countries, adolescent girls are being infected with HIV at a rate five or more times higher than boys.

p. 31 A young couple talks under the glow of a street light. Biologically, a woman's risk of acquiring sexually transmitted infections during unprotected sexual relations is two to four times that of men. Younger women are at greater risk because their reproductive tracts are still maturing.

p. 32 Actors teach villagers about the dangers of AIDS and what can be done to prevent it, in Fidel Castro Village of Mozambique. Groups like this one provide information about rights and prevention by mixing contemporary messages with traditional teaching methods, such as theater and dance.

p. 33 Roselane Madubedube (left) is one of twin brides, marrying husband Ignatius Sefafe Mokhomo. Her sister, Rose Mabale

Seqhomoko and new husband William are also in the photograph, taken at their double wedding in Maputsoe, Lesotho.

grave. Flowers are placed in the dirt, but they are broken first to discourage vendors who sell flowers at the cemetery from coming back to steal them for resale, a common practice.

pp. 66, 67 Karabo Docus Tlebere died at just 9 months of age. Mother Patricia Tlebere and grandmother Christina Tlebere sit in the house with the coffin of the young child and then at the burial site. This was the third child lost by mother Patricia; two previous children were stillborn.

p. 68 Children near Maseru, Lesoth, persevere against the wind and rain after school.

p. 69 Mamello Mokholokoe, herself physically challenged after a leg operation, created Phelisanong, a community-based project to rehabilitate, educate and train disabled children and youth. They provide HIV education, support groups and outreach for orphans and other vulnerable children. Mamello holds orphan Mamakhooa Maeketsi, 8, while Setlehko Moti, 7, touches her cheek. See Call To Action.

p. 70 Malihlahleng Rathebe is a grandmother raising seven grandchildren, five of whom are in this picture. According to helpage.org, as the AIDS pandemic continues large percentages of older people are left caring for orphans and vulnerable children. Older people are some of the poorest, and HIV/AIDS exacerbates the extreme poverty faced by households of the elderly.

p. 71 Flory Kolobe is surrounded by some of the 80 orphans in her program. Tsepong Counseling Centre was established in 2001 to raise HIV/AIDS awareness in both rural and urban areas. It helps provide counseling services and HIV testing at the Senkatana Clinic Centre while supporting orphans and vulnerable children. See Call to Action.

pp. 72, 73 Children play in the schoolyard of the Early Childhood Education Center School in Harare, Ethiopia. Education and the affordability of school fees are a major issue for those countries that charge fees for students' education, since many parents cannot afford the money to send their children to school. Fees can amount to almost one-

third of the income of poorer families. School fees are also one of the biggest barriers to the adoption of AIDS orphans.

p. 74 5-year-old Shito Redo was due to have a female circumcision performed on the day this photo was taken near Harare, Ethiopia. It was called off after her parents reconsidered. Community activists from the Professional Alliance For Development in Ethiopia are trying to educate villagers about harmful traditional practices.

p. 75 Communities are fighting to prevent the abduction of young girls. Tedule Segut, 16, (left) and Heseret Hurade, 15, are from Iluitaya, Ethiopia. These two girls were abducted on different days, but quick-thinking villagers rescued both girls before they were assaulted. Community leaders are trying to raise awareness to help stop this from happening.

p. 76 A boy and his grandmother photographed at their home, near Harare, Ethiopia. There were an estimated 539,000 AIDS orphans (children having lost one or both parents) in Ethiopia in 2003; a cumulative total of 90,000 adults and 25,000 children had died of AIDS by the end of 2003.

p. 77 A group of children pose for a photograph in Leribe, Lesotho. An estimated 12 million children under the age of 17 (just under 10% of all children) living in sub-Saharan Africa have lost one or both parents to AIDS.

p. 78 Young girls play at Tsakholo Primary School outside of Maseru, Lesotho. In 2005, sub-Saharan Africa was home to 2 million children under 15 years of age living with HIV.

p. 79 Boys play soccer at a cemetery in Harare, Ethiopia. Almost 90% of the total number of children with HIV are living in sub-Saharan Africa. Fewer than one in ten of those children are being reached by basic support services.

p. 80 Free condom dispensers, Lesotho. UNFPA, the largest public-sector purchaser of male condoms, estimates the global supply of public-sector condoms is less than 50% of that need-

ed to ensure adequate condom coverage. The agency estimates that the gap between supply and actual need totals 8.3 billion condoms.

p. 81 *Left:* Mapalesa Selia-lia has been a nurse clinician for more than 30 years. On this day at the Mahobong Health Clinic she saw 57 patients from nearby villages. She does AIDS testing and counseling as well as treating whatever comes her way. Here she listens to a fetal heartbeat.
Right: Near Vilankulos, Mozambique: weight at birth is a good indicator not only of a mother's health and nutritional status, but also of the newborn's chances for survival, growth, long-term health and psychosocial development.

pp. 82-83 Peace Corps volunteer Jean Margaritis Otto and youth counselor Tsepo Rameane (not pictured) discuss HIV and AIDS with students from grades 8 through 10 at Mahobong Secondary School in Leribe, Lesotho. Students are taught how to open condoms, how to properly use them and to check expiration dates. The school has 130 students; 60-70% of the students are either single or double orphans.

p. 84 Tenth-grade students giggle as they hold a condom in their classroom. From left: Majobo Mapesnoane, 16; Limakatso Romajake, 16; and Ronsang Rakobuoa, 16. Contrary to common fears or stereotypes, extensive research has detected little evidence that sex education leads to an increase in sexual activity.

p. 85 Boys react to a condom filled with air on their desk at Mahobong Secondary School. To ensure a sufficient condom supply and to halt the AIDS epidemic by 2015, the level of funding for condom procurement and distribution needs to triple.

p. 86 Fusi Matli, 11, a fourth-grade student at English Grammar School in Teyateyaneng, Lesotho, eats coco berries near his home after school.

p. 87 Clothes dry on the branches of a tree outside Maseru, Lesotho.

p. 88 This is a view from a car window near Leribe, Lesotho. Lesotho is a small, moun-

tainous, landlocked country situated entirely within the borders of South Africa.

p. 89 The red ribbon is the global symbol of solidarity uniting people in the common fight against HIV/AIDS. According to The Red Ribbon Foundation, red, like love, is a symbol of passion and tolerance towards those affected; like blood, red also represents the pain caused by deaths from AIDS. Red symbolizes anger over the helplessness we sometimes encounter fighting a disease for which there is still no cure. Finally, red is a sign of warning against one of the biggest problems of our time.

p. 90 Peace Corps volunteer Jean Margaritis Otto holds the hand of Letuta Mofoleng, 46, while fellow volunteer Leigh Marrero comforts her. Mr. Mofoleng died the next day.

p. 92 A suggestion box at one of the government buildings in Maseru, Lesotho.

p. 93 James Moama, 33, at the Mother of Mercy Hospice in Chilanga, just outside Lusaka, Zambia. Sub-Saharan Africa remains the worst affected region for AIDS in the world. In 2005, there were 24.5 million people in sub-Saharan Africa living with HIV. Globally, 64% of all people living with HIV live in sub-Saharan Africa.

Acknowledgements

I started this project with an assignment from Andrew Stawicki, Peter Robertson and the crew from PhotoSensitive in Africa: Patti Gower, Peter Bregg, Dick Loek, V. Tony Hauser, Bernard Weil and Care Canada. I thank them for bringing me to Africa and igniting my passion for this continent and this story, which I will continue to follow.

To Giuseppe Liverani and Francesca Sorace whose compassion and social conscience made this project come to life. Also thanks to Filomena Moscatelli, Daniela Meda, and the staff of Charta in Milan.

Lucas Robinson, thank you for your research, friendship and help. To Jean Margaritis Otto, who inspired me with her passion and care for people combined with a fiery determination to make things better. To Patrick Reed, Oscar Reed, Ao Loo, John Westheuser, and the people at White Pine Pictures who created the exceptional documentary *Tsepong: A Clinic Called Hope*.

To my friends, colleagues and family who encouraged and helped me to do this project.

Jamie White, Chuck Kuehn, Alicia Homer, Philip Berger, Christina Magill, Stephen Lewis, Seraanye Selialia, Mathabisang Leputla, Kenny and Tsepo, Lesotho Funeral Services, Bree Seeley, Frank Madden, Beau Madden, Rita Leistner, Katja Heinemann, Jason Eskenazi, Marc Rochette, Lesley Sparks, Andy Clark, Stephanie Nolan, Kathy Sperberg, Pierre Vachon, Erin Elder, Antonio DeLuca, Chris Diemert, Ethan Eisenberg, Ben Rondel, Yuri Dojc, Shannon Eckstein, Kirsten Rian, Sara Terry, Brian Howell, Mauro Fiorese, John Trotter, Christine Ryan, Morgan Broman, Mike Petro, Rachel Pilliod, Osvaldo, Alvaro, Oklahoma Arts Institute, Derek Jennings, Robin Huston, Jeanne Parkhurst, Conrad Eek, Ben Long, Eric Foss, David Friend, Jean Francois Leroy, Kathy Ryan, Sarah Barton, Chloe Sherman, Jay DeFoore, Tom Mayenknecht, Michael Regnier, Andre Chitayat, David Schonauer, Darren Ching, Bono, Candida, Kate, Katrina, Edith Mohapi, M.D. Kathy Ferrer, Refiloe Mpholo, Doris Magdalinski, Jesse Moore, Jessica Nelligan, Jennifer Young, Russell Armstrong, Marnie Mitchel, Makhosi Fosa-Serobe, Masenate Matsolo, Nkeletseng Kanetsi, Julian Rademeyer, Kassa Rorissa, Betigel Workalemahu, Phil Maher, Jill Sloan, Biruk Abebe, Tesfu, Joy Sun, Denise Thomas, Paddy Fay, Barbaara Nkoala, Susan Bruckner, Eric Thehane, Ms. Brown, Moses Marshall, Alex Sekikila, Flore Kolobe, Mamello Mokholokoe, Ben Mokholokoe, Miriam Mamotete, Hmanuel Mekonnen, Tesfu Mlagata, Andrea Palframan, Gary McNutt, Charity Chinama, Kate Greenaway, Barbara Lopi, Margaret Li, Janice Dawe, Laura Blaney, Juliet Lyon, Erica Heiman, Claudio Quefass, Avery Lozada, Gallery One, Laurel Fischtein, Goldie Konopny, Sharon Fischtein, Kevin Willson, Jennifer Konopny, Juan Travnik, Bob Todrick, Joel Breslof, Judy Anderson, Larry Anderson, The Marcus Family, Frances Simon, Teresa Simon and Barry Kirsh.

To Tanja Rohweder, whose patience, love and understanding, along with her endless encouragement to pursue this story, helped make it happen. And to the countless Heroines and Heroes I have met and photographed in my travels through Africa.

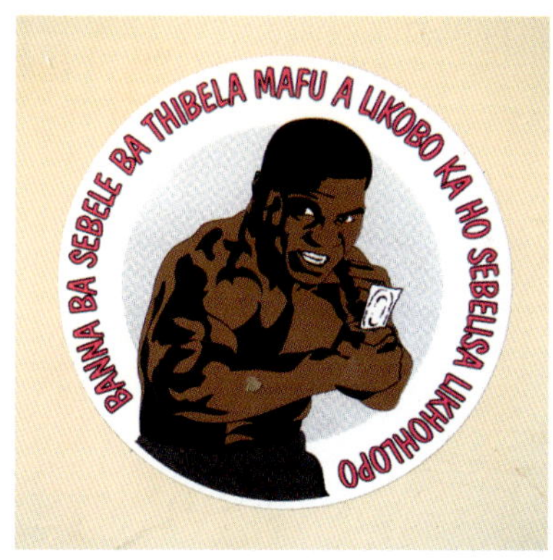

To find out more about Charta,
and to learn about our most recent publications, visit

www.chartaartbooks.it

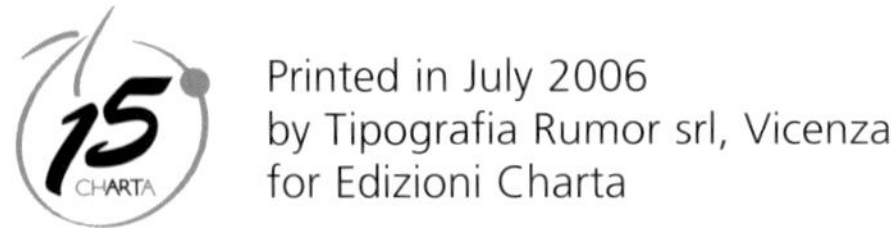

Printed in July 2006
by Tipografia Rumor srl, Vicenza
for Edizioni Charta